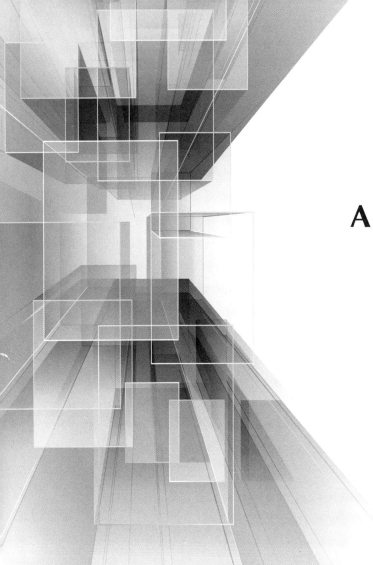

A Competency-Based Framework for Health Education Specialists – 2015

Copyright 2015.
The National Commission for Health Education Credentialing, Inc.
and the Society for Public Health Education, Inc.

All rights reserved. ISBN 978-0-9652570-7-7

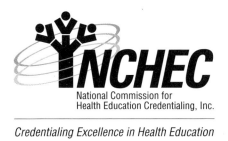
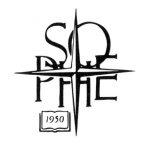

A Competency-Based Framework for Health Education Specialists – 2015

For reprint permission or ordering information contact:
The National Commission for Health Education Credentialing, Inc.
1541 Alta Drive, Suite 303 Whitehall, PA 18052-5642 www.nchec.org 888-624-3248.

Suggested Citation: National Commission for Health Education Credentialing, Inc. & Society for Public Health Education. (2015). *A competency-based framework for health education specialists - 2015. Whitehall, PA: Author.*

Acknowledgements

Health Education Specialist Practice Analysis 2015 Contributors

A qualified, competent health workforce is an essential element in efforts to improve the public's health. The health education profession has contributed to this goal since the 1970s by undertaking rigorous scientific efforts to identify Competencies that reflect the knowledge and skills needed by health education specialists in all practice settings. This National Health Education Specialist Practice Analysis 2015 (HESPA 2015) Model represents the latest evolution of Health Education Competencies, which underlie the profession's commitment to excellence in health education teaching, research, and practice.

The National Commission for Health Education Credentialing, Inc. (NCHEC) and the Society for Public Health Education, Inc. (SOPHE) are proud to lead the health education profession in sponsoring the HESPA research and publishing this document as well as its companion, *The HESPA 2015 Technical Report*. SOPHE and NCHEC are the joint copyright holders of these publications and the research data.

We recognize that an initiative of this breadth and depth would not be possible without the expertise and dedication of many individuals. First, we extend our deep appreciation to Dixie Dennis, PhD, MCHES, and James F. McKenzie, PhD, MPH, MCHES, who, as co-chairs of the HESPA 2015 Task Force, devoted thousands of hours to guiding the project's conceptualization, implementation, data analysis, and interpretation. Their extensive knowledge of the health education profession, research skills, leadership, and perseverance helped move the project forward in a scientifically rigorous and timely fashion. Second, sincere thanks goes to Carla M. Caro, MA, and Patricia M. Muenzen, MA, of the Professional Examination Service (ProExam) of New York, a nonprofit credentialing and competency assurance organization contracted to assist with the HESPA 2015 project. We are indebted to their proficiency, professionalism, and devotion to this project as well as to the advancement of the health education profession.

On a broader scale, our gratitude extends to many other volunteers whose names are listed on the next page and who served in various roles related to study procedures and/or the development of this publication. Last but not least, we appreciate the thousands of health education specialists who voluntarily completed the HESPA 2015 survey, as well as hundreds of professional volunteers who contributed to the work described in this book. All those who assisted in HESPA 2015 can take pride in helping pave the way for a health education workforce that is knowledgeable and skilled in the face of today's health challenges.

Linda Lysoby, MS, MCHES, CAE,
Executive Director, NCHEC

M. Elaine Auld, MPH, MCHES,
Chief Executive Officer, SOPHE

Acknowledgements

Contributors to *A Competency-Based Framework for Health Education Specialists – 2015*

Editors
James F. McKenzie, PhD, MPH, MCHES
Dixie Dennis, PhD, MCHES

Contributing Authors
Kelly Brennan, MEd, MCHES
Randall R. Cottrell, DEd, MCHES
Eva I. Doyle, PhD, MCHES
Jenni Flanagan, BS, CHES
Michele Guadalupe, MPH
Cynthia S. Kusorgbor-Narh, MPH, CHES
Denise M. Seabert, PhD, MCHES
Starr Wharton, MS, MCHES

Reviewers
M. Elaine Auld, MPH, MCHES
Carla M. Caro, MA
Linda Lysoby, MS, MCHES, CAE
Patricia M. Muenzen, MA
Melissa Opp, MPH, MCHES
Jacquie Rainey, DrPH, MCHES
Laura Rasar King, MPH, MCHES
Alyson Taub, EdD, MCHES
Alexis M. Williams, MPH, MS, CHES

Copy Editor
Caitlin Rizzo

Table of Contents

Acknowledgements iii
List of Contributors iv
Table of Contents v
List of Tables vii
List of Figures viii
Introduction ix
Section I: Historical Perspectives 1
    Role Delineation 1
    Professional Preparation and Certification 1
    Graduate-Level Areas of Responsibility, Competencies, and Sub-competencies 2
    Competences Update Project (CUP) 2
    Health Educator Job Analysis 2010 (HEJA 2010) 3
    Implications of Revalidation of Competencies Studies on Individual Certification .4
    Accreditation of the CHES and MCHES Certification Program 5
    Competency-Based Accreditation 5
    Moving Forward: Continued Growth and Change 7
Section II: HESPA 2015 Process and Outcomes 9
    HESPA 2015 Participants 9
    HESPA 2015 Procedures 10
        Conceptual Framework for Instrument Development 12
        Survey Instrument 13
    Analysis and Outcomes 14
        Demographics 14
        Generic Sub-competencies 20
        Entry- and Advanced-level Sub-competencies 20
        Refinement and Finalization of the Framework 21
        The Validated Model 22
        Verified Knowledge Items 24
    Discussion 24
        Validated Areas of Responsibilities, Competencies, and Sub-competencies 24
        Verified Knowledge Items 25
    Summary 26
Section III: The HESPA 2015 Model 27
    Area I: Assess Needs, Resources, and Capacity for Health Education/Promotion ..29
    Area II: Plan Health Education/Promotion 34
    Area III: Implement Health Education/Promotion 39
    Area IV: Conduct Evaluation and Research Related to Health Education/Promotion .43
    Area V: Administer and Manage Health Education/Promotion 49
    Area VI: Serve as a Health Education/Promotion Resource Person 55
    Area VII: Communicate, Promote, and Advocate for
        Health, Health Education/Promotion, and the Profession 59

Table of Contents

Section IV: Using the HESPA 2015 Model 65
    Health Education Students 65
    College and University Faculty Members 65
    Health Education Practitioners 66
    Professional Development Providers 66
    Other Health Professionals 66
    Health Education Employers 66
    Leaders of Professional Credentialing and Program Accreditation 67
    Policy Makers and Funding Agencies 67
    Recommendations to the Profession 67

Section V: Changes in the Areas of Responsibility, Competencies, and Sub-competencies 69
of Health Education Specialists from 1985 to 2015
    Seven Areas of Responsibility 69
    Competencies and Sub-competencies 71
    Area I: Assess Needs, Resources, and Capacity for Health Education/Promotion 72
    Area II: Plan Health Education/Promotion 73
    Area III: Implement Health Education/Promotion 73
    Area IV: Conduct Evaluation and Research Related to Health Education/Promotion 73
    Area V: Administer and Manage Health Education/Promotion 74
    Area VI: Serve as a Health Education/Promotion Resource Person 75
    Area VII: Communicate, Promote, and Advocate for Health, Health Education/
        Promotion, and the Profession 75

Section VI: Core Knowledge Items 77

References 85

Appendix A: Glossary 89

Appendix B: Comparison of the Competencies and Sub-competencies of the
    HEJA 2010 Model and the HESPA 2015 Model 91

    Appendix B1: Comparison of the Competencies, and Sub-competencies of the
        HEJA 2010 Model and the HESPA 2015 Model 92

    Appendix B2: Comparison of the Competencies and Sub-competencies of the
        HESPA 2015 Model and the HEJA 2010 Model 105

Appendix C: History of Working Groups for Health Education Specialist 119
Competency Development

Appendix D: Competency Matrices 123
    Directions for Use of the Area of Responsibility Matrices 123
    Directions for Use of the Analysis Sheets 125
    Purpose of the Matrices and Analysis Sheets 127
    Adapting Existing Curricula 127
    Developing New Curricula 129
    Selecting Teaching-Learning Strategies 129
    The Competency Framework by Areas of Responsibility 129

List of Tables

Table 2.1.	Demographic Data of Survey Participants	15
Table 2.2.	Professional Data of Survey Participants	17
Table 2.3.	Work Settings of Survey Participants	19
Table 3.1.	Health Education Specialist Practice Analysis 2015 Model: Overview of Areas of Responsibilities and Competencies	27
Table 3.2.	Health Education Specialist Practice Analysis 2015 Model: Area I: Assess Needs, Resources, and Capacity for Health Education/Promotion	31
Table 3.3.	Health Education Specialist Practice Analysis 2015 Model: Area II: Plan Health Education/Promotion	36
Table 3.4.	Health Education Specialist Practice Analysis 2015 Model: Area III: Implement Health Education/Promotion	41
Table 3.5.	Health Education Specialist Practice Analysis 2015 Model: Area IV: Conduct Evaluation and Research Related to Health Education/Promotion	45
Table 3.6.	Health Education Specialist Practice Analysis 2015 Model: Area V: Administer and Manage Health Education/Promotion	51
Table: 3.7.	Health Education Specialist Practice Analysis 2015 Model: Area VI: Serve as a Health Education/Promotion Resource Person	57
Table 3.8.	Health Education Specialist Practice Analysis 2015 Model: Area VII: Communicate, Promote, and Advocate for Health, Health Education/ Promotion, and the Profession	61
Table 5.1.	Comparison of Areas of Responsibility (1985 - 2015)	70
Table 5.2.	Competencies and Sub-competencies at Each Level of Practice between the HEJA 2010 and the HESPA 2015 Models	72
Table 6.1.	Validated Knowledge Items by Topic and Area of Responsibility	78
Table B.1.	Comparison of HEJA 2010 Model (Old) and HESPA 2015 (New): *The HEJA 2010 Model* (Old) Perspective	93
Table B.2.	Comparison of HESPA 2015 Model (New) and HEJA 2010 (Old): *The HESPA 2015 Model* (New) Perspective	105

List of Figures

Figure 1.1.	Historical Timeline of Selected Milestones	8
Figure 2.1.	HESPA 2015 Process	11
Figure D.1.	Example Area of Responsibility Matrix Analysis	124
Figure D.2.	Example Analysis Sheet for the Areas of Responsibility	126
Figure D.3.	Sample Questions for Curriculum Decision-Making	128
Figure D.4.	Area of Responsibility I Matrix	130
Figure D.5.	Area of Responsibility II Matrix	131
Figure D.6.	Area of Responsibility III Matrix	132
Figure D.7.	Area of Responsibility IV Matrix	133
Figure D.7.A.	Area IV: Advanced 2-level—Part A Matrix	134
Figure D.7.B.	Area IV: Advanced 2-level—Part B Matrix	134
Figure D.8.	Area of Responsibility V Matrix	135
Figure D.9.	Area of Responsibility VI Matrix	136
Figure D.10.	Area of Responsibility VII Matrix	137
Figure D.11.	Analysis Sheet: Areas of Responsibility, Entry-level	138
Figure D.12.	Analysis Sheet: Areas of Responsibility, Advanced 1-level	139
Figure D.13.	Analysis Sheet: Areas of Responsibility, Advanced 2-level	140

Introduction

The purpose of this publication is to communicate the Responsibilities, Competencies, and Sub-competencies that are essential to contemporary health education/promotion practice. This document contains descriptions of the processes, outcomes, and related materials of the most recent update project known as the Health Education Specialist Practice Analysis 2015 (HESPA 2015). This Model is designed for use by those in the health education/promotion profession as a framework for professional preparation, credentialing, and professional development.

Section I of this document contains a brief overview of historical perspectives related to the growth and evolution of the health education/promotion profession and its quality assurance efforts. In Section II, the processes and outcomes of HESPA 2015 are described. In Section III, the resulting HESPA 2015 Model containing the updated Areas of Responsibility, Competencies, and Sub-competencies for health education specialists is presented. Section IV contains recommended uses of the HESPA 2015 Model for various stakeholders and a set of seven specific recommendations for the profession. Section V provides a comparison of the HESPA 2015 Model with the Health Educator Job Analysis 2010 (HEJA 2010) Model. Section VI includes a set of knowledge items verified in the HESPA 2015 analysis as useful in the practice of health education/promotion. The appendices include additional materials that can be used to master professional terminology and adapt professional preparation and development efforts to the HESPA 2015.

This page was
intentionally left blank

Section I: Historical Perspectives

The HESPA 2015 Model continues the historically strong vision among health education specialists to embrace contemporary practice and lead others into the future. The historical perspectives below serve as evidence of this pioneering spirit. This section contains an overview of the first role delineation project and its impact on professional preparation programs and certification, the development of graduate-level Areas of Responsibility, Competencies, and Sub- competencies, the development of the Competencies Update Project (CUP) Model, which led to three levels of practice defined by years of experience and educational degree, and the use of best practice job analysis methods that led to the development of the HEJA 2010 Model.

This section also contains information about a series of accreditation task forces that worked to lay the foundation for high quality professional preparation and practice standards in health education and strategic directions for program accreditation and individual credentialing.

Role Delineation

The history of health education in the United States dates back to the late 19th century with the establishment of the first academic programs preparing school health educators (Allegrante et al., 2004). In the 1940s, interest in quality assurance and the development of standards for professional preparation of health educators became aligned. Over the next several decades, professional associations produced guidelines for preparing health educators and introduced accreditation efforts. Yet, it was not until the 1970s that health education began evolving as a true profession (Livingood & Auld, 2001). In addition to defining a body of literature, health education professional organizations began to promulgate a Health Education Code of Ethics, as well as agree upon the use of terminology, a skill-based set of Competencies, rigorous systems for quality assurance, and a health education credentialing system.

Long standing questions about the practice of health educators eventually led to the first Role Delineation Project in the 1970s. In February 1978, health educators from all practice settings assembled at the First Bethesda Conference to begin the process of defining and verifying their role. The stated purposes of the conference were: (a) to analyze the commonalities and differences that existed in the preparation of health educators within different practice settings and (b) to determine the potential for developing acceptable guidelines for professional preparation that would include all practice settings (NCHEC, 1985). The conference attendees recommended the establishment of the National Task Force on the Preparation and Practice of Health Educators, and this recommendation was realized in March 1978. In collaboration with the National Center for Health Education, this task force undertook the landmark Role Delineation Project (United States Department of Health, Education, and Welfare, 1978).

Following considerable public discussion and background research, the Role Delineation Project resulted in the role of entry-level health educators during the years 1978 to 1981. After conducting a national survey of practicing health educators, which helped verify and define the role of the health educator, the leaders of that project concluded that there was a "generic role" common to all health educators. That is, commonalities in the roles and functions of entry-level health educators existed regardless of whether they were employed in schools, communities, health care facilities, worksites, or other settings. This finding formed the basis for health education credentialing and the refinement of academic programs in health education.

Professional Preparation and Certification

Between 1981 and 1985, the National Task Force on the Preparation and Practice of Health Educators developed a curriculum framework using the defined role. This framework was based on contributions from academics and practitioners

Section I: Historical Perspectives

involved in two national conferences, several regional workshops, and many meetings of professional associations. The resulting document, *A Framework for the Development of Competency-Based Curricula for Entry-Level Health Educators* (NCHEC, 1985), provided individuals associated with professional preparation programs a frame of reference for developing or refining a health education curriculum. A Competency was defined as the "...ability to apply a certain specified skill in dealing with some defined amount of meaningful subject matter" (NCHEC, 1985, p. 2). As such, the framework included Competencies as a reflection of both content and process.

During the Second Bethesda Conference in 1986, attendees reached a consensus that a certification process was appropriate to ensure that individuals delivering health education services possessed a minimal level of competence. Preliminary steps for developing a national certification system for health educators were initiated, culminating with the establishment of the National Commission for Health Education Credentialing, Inc. (NCHEC) in 1988. Following a charter certification phase in 1989, during which individuals who met eligibility requirements could become certified through a review of documentation submitted (e.g., letters of support, academic records), the NCHEC offered the first national Competency-based certification examination in 1990. Thus, the results of this role delineation process formed the basis for a: (a) framework for professional preparation, (b) national examination, leading to credentialing the eligible individuals as Certified Health Education Specialists (CHES), and (c) guide for continuing education for practitioners (NCHEC, 1996).

Graduate-Level Areas of Responsibility, Competencies, and Sub-competencies

In 1992, the American Association for Health Education (AAHE) and the Society for Public Health Education (SOPHE) initiated efforts to determine graduate-level Areas of Responsibility, Competencies, and Sub-competencies when they commissioned the Joint Committee for Graduate Standards (AAHE, NCHEC, & SOPHE, 1999). The committee sought the input of individuals involved in graduate-level professional preparation through a national survey and at various annual professional associations' meetings, as well as its own continuing deliberations, to ascertain the advanced-level of practice by health educators with advanced training and experience. The committee projected that its work would build on the entry-level skills within the Seven Areas of Responsibility already identified, as well as establish new Areas of Responsibility at the advanced-levels.

Following the publication of a final report and its acceptance by the boards of AAHE, NCHEC, and SOPHE, the Graduate Competencies Implementation Committee was formed (SOPHE & AAHE, 1997). Committee members addressed the manner in which the new advanced-level Areas of Responsibility, Competencies, and Sub-competencies would be disseminated to, and implemented by, the profession. The resulting document, *A Competency-Based Framework for Graduate-Level Health Educators,* was jointly published by AAHE, NCHEC, and SOPHE (1999). This publication also contained a history of the work of the Committee.

Competencies Update Project (CUP)

During the mid-to-late 1990s, professional organizations and individual health educators expressed a desire to reverify the role of entry-level health educators to ensure that it reflected the then contemporary practice and to further develop, refine, and validate the role of advanced-level health educators. To accomplish this, NCHEC initiated the National Health Educator Competencies Update Project (CUP) in 1998 with the participation of AAHE, SOPHE, and nine other national health education related organizations. This multiphase national research study was guided by the CUP National Advisory

Section I: Historical Perspectives

Committee, consisting of representatives of the 12 national professional groups and a three-person CUP Steering Committee that led the project with assistance from research experts (Gilmore, Olsen, Taub, & Connell, 2005). The project included a planning and resource development phase (1998-1999), a survey development and pilot process phase (2000-2001), and a four-year data collection, analysis, and reporting phase (2001-2004).

An updated model that included Seven Areas of Responsibility, 35 Competencies, and 163 Sub-competencies emerged from the study (Gilmore et al., 2005). The CUP Hierarchical Model identified three levels of practice, each building on the other, defined by years of experience and degrees:
- *entry-level:* less than five years of experience with a baccalaureate or master's degree
- *advanced 1-level:* five or more years of experience with a baccalaureate or master's degree
- *advanced 2-level:* five or more years of experience with a doctoral degree

Based on statistical analyses and professional judgment, the CUP Hierarchical Model emerged with implications for professional preparation, credentialing, and professional development (Gilmore et al., 2005). A new edition of *A Competency-Based Framework for Health Educators* (NCHEC, SOPHE, & AAHE, 2006) was published based on the CUP results.

In addition to that publication in 2005, SOPHE, AAHE, and NCHEC issued four recommendations that were unanimously endorsed in 2006 by the Coalition of National Health Education Organizations (CNHEO), a coalition of professional organizations of which health education specialists are members. These recommendations included preparing students in baccalaureate and graduate programs to perform all Seven Areas of Responsibility with baccalaureate students expected to master the entry-level, and graduate students expected to master entry- and advanced-level Competencies and Sub-competencies of the CUP Model. In addition, the recommendations included that NCHEC base the entry-level certification examination on entry-level components of the CUP Model (Airhihenbuwa et al., 2005).

Health Educator Job Analysis 2010 (HEJA 2010)
To keep the description of the practice of health education specialists contemporary and to meet the accreditation standards of the National Commission for Certifying Agencies (NCCA) (see the "Accreditation of the CHES and MCHES Certification Programs" section of this publication for more information on accreditation of credentials), the HEJA study was launched in 2008 and completed in 2009. Job analysis experts from Professional Examination Service (ProExam) helped design and guide the study. These ProExam experts partnered with a five-member steering committee (chief staff officers of NCHEC, SOPHE, and AAHE, the 2008 coordinator of the NCHEC Division Board for Certification of Health Education Specialists, and the appointed HEJA task force chair), an 11-member task force, and 49 volunteer subject matter experts, independent reviewers, and survey pilot participants to carry out the work.

The multiphase, national, 18-month HEJA study entailed two general phases: (a) instrument development and (b) implementation (i.e., data collection and analysis). The instrument development phase included in-depth interviews of subject matter experts, independent reviews by representatives of diverse health education work settings, and a modified Delphi approach through which task force members systematically integrated the interview and review outcomes into the instrument development process. A pilot survey resulted in further instrument refinement prior to the launch of the online survey. An updated model that included Seven Areas of

Section I: Historical Perspectives

Responsibility, 34 Competencies, and 223 Sub-competencies emerged from the study (NCHEC, SOPHE, & AAHE, 2010). The three distinct levels of practice established through the CUP study were reverified in the HEJA study. As was the case in the CUP study, the HEJA 2010 Model emerged based on extensive statistical analysis and professional judgment. This HEJA Model included a hierarchy of entry-, advanced 1-, and advanced 2-level Sub-competencies.

Similar to the CUP study, the HEJA 2010 Steering Committee made recommendations for implementation of the HEJA results. The CNHEO and the National Implementation Task Force for Accreditation in Health Education endorsed those recommendations. The steering committee recommended that: (a) appropriate levels of Sub-competencies be used in professional preparation programs, (b) NCHEC use the entry-level Sub-competencies for the CHES certification examination, (c) NCHEC use both the entry- and advanced-level Sub-competencies for the certification examination for the new Master Certified Health Education Specialist (MCHES) credential, and (d) all Sub-competencies be used for professional development activities.

Implications of Revalidation of Competencies Studies on Individual Certification

The results of previous studies (i.e., the CUP and HEJA 2010 Models) that have revalidated Competencies have had an impact on individual certification. The dissemination and endorsement of the CUP Model initiated changes to the structure of the CHES examination for entry-level health education specialists and discussions about the possible need for an advanced-level certification. NCHEC leaders updated the CHES examination blueprint framework for the certification examination questions, released a new study guide (NCHEC, 2007), and launched the first CHES examination based on the CUP Model in the fall of 2007. Performance pass rates on the new examination were comparable to previous performance pass rates (Dennis & Mahoney, 2008). These comparable performance pass rates validated beliefs that the primary components of the CUP Model not only reflected contemporary practice but also the professional preparation programs that are often shaped by contemporary practice.

CUP findings regarding advanced-levels of practice held significant implications for NCHEC and the profession. The results of an NCHEC sponsored survey of stakeholders, and further discussions with multiple national leadership groups also supported moving ahead. Additionally, creating distinct levels of certification aligned with the recommendations of the National Task Force on Accreditation in Health Education (Allegrante et al., 2004). These factors and feasibility deliberations among various NCHEC working groups led NCHEC leaders to announce plans to develop an advanced-level of certification in the fall of 2008. In May 2009 following a period of public comment about such issues as eligibility criteria and certification mechanisms, the NCHEC Board of Commissioners issued a policy statement regarding a new advanced-level credential (NCHEC, 2009). This statement revealed the name of the certification was Master Certified Health Education Specialist (MCHES) and included that eligibility for MCHES was five years of experience, with certification based on a combination of entry- and advanced-level Competencies and Sub-competencies.

Following the completion of the HEJA 2010 Model confirming an updated model of entry- and advanced-levels, the results were used to create a revised examination for CHES. The advanced-level Competencies were first used in the Experience Documentation Opportunity (2010-2011) for current CHES, which led to the MCHES credential first being awarded in April 2011 (NCHEC, 2010a). The inaugural MCHES examination was administered in October 2011. The results of HEJA 2010 also were used to establish professional development standards for those holding the MCHES credential.

Accreditation of the CHES and MCHES Certification Programs

In the midst of developments toward advanced-level certification, NCHEC leaders also decided to engage in accreditation efforts specific to entry-level certification. In June 2008, the CHES certification program was granted accreditation by the National Commission for Certifying Agencies (NCCA), the accreditation body of the Institute for Credentialing Excellence (ICE) that accredits professional certification organizations (ICE, 2009). Obtaining the initial recognition of CHES by this leading body in testing accreditation made a profound statement within the national credentialing industry about the quality of the CHES examination and its reflection of a clearly defined profession (NCHEC, 2008). In May 2013, the CHES certification was granted reaccreditation, and the MCHES certification was granted accreditation in its first review.

Critical to the progress of the health education profession is that, among the NCCA *Standards for the Accreditation of Certification Programs*, it is required that a professional role delineation or job analysis be conducted and periodically validated (ICE, 2009). To ensure that the content of NCHEC examinations reflects current practice in the profession and meets certification program accreditation standards, NCHEC committed to conducting job analyses every five years. In keeping with the five-year cycle, after HEJA 2010, the HESPA 2015 began in February 2013 and concluded in August 2014.

Competency-Based Academic Program Accreditation

Various issues facing the profession in quality assurance, including a fragmented system of program approval processes and accreditation mechanisms, were addressed in 2000 by AAHE and SOPHE with an invitational meeting of key health education leaders. As a result, the National Task Force on Accreditation in Heath Education was convened by AAHE and SOPHE from 2001 to 2003 and charged with developing a detailed plan for a coordinated accreditation system for baccalaureate and graduate programs in health education. The Task Force's findings and recommendation laid the foundation for high quality professional preparation and practice standards in health education and provided strategic directions related to accreditation of community and school heath education pre-service programs and also provided strategic direction for individual credentialing (Allegrante et al., 2004).

A critical recommendation from the meeting was that "a comprehensive, coordinated accreditation system for undergraduate and graduate health education should be put into place, which builds on the strengths of current mechanisms" (Allegrante et al., 2004, p. 672). Subsequently, between 2001 and 2003 the National Task Force on Accreditation in Health Education developed principles and seven recommendations for strengthening both professional preparation and certification in health education. In 2004, AAHE and SOPHE commissioned a new task force, the National Transition Task Force on Accreditation in Health Education, to help implement the recommendations between 2004 and 2006. In 2006, this task force convened in Dallas, Texas, for the Third National Congress for Institutions Preparing Health Educators, a landmark meeting sometimes referred to as Dallas II. This conference was referred to as Dallas II because the earlier congress of 1996, which was designed for attendees to discuss graduate-level Competencies, was also held in Dallas (the first congress was in Birmingham, Alabama, in 1981) (Taub, Birch, Auld, Lysoby, & Rasar King, 2009).

Section I: Historical Perspectives

The Dallas II meeting, sponsored by SOPHE and AAHE, drew together approximately 250 university faculty members and administrators from over 150 professional preparation programs (Taub et al., 2009), as well as practitioners. The purpose of Dallas II was to provide an update of the effort to establish a unified system of accreditation for the health education profession, review and discuss future accreditation developments, disseminate and discuss the implications of the new CUP Model, and identify issues and strategies for the transition to a unified accreditation system.

According to Taub et al. (2009), accreditation discussions focused on potential avenues for transitioning to a more coordinated system. Since 1988, AAHE had partnered with the National Council for Accreditation of Teacher Education (NCATE), the officially recognized accrediting body for professional preparation programs in school health education. The Council on Education for Public Health (CEPH) had been accrediting master's level programs and schools of public health since 1974 (a process originally established and maintained by the American Public Health Association since the early 1940s). In 1980, SOPHE established an approval process for baccalaureate public or community health education programs, and in 1984 AAHE joined to form the SOPHE/AAHE Baccalaureate Program Approval Committee (SABPAC). SABPAC approval was based on the Competencies of health education specialists and included a peer-review process based on self-study using assessment criteria. However, the lack of an official accreditation designation for the SABPAC was a challenge. In 2005, CEPH began to accredit baccalaureate public or community health education programs linked to graduate public health programs and schools, but did not accredit standalone baccalaureate public or community health education programs (CEPH, 2005).

A part of the Dallas II discussions revolved around the possibility of CEPH becoming the accrediting body for all professional preparation programs in community health education, regardless of their affiliation status with graduate-level public health schools and programs (Taub et al., 2009). Attendees discussed challenges as they related to differences in terminology regarding a "unified" versus a "coordinated" multiple body accrediting system, potential philosophical differences between public and community health, and capacity challenges for small professional preparation programs that needed to be accredited.

Dallas II attendees deemed further exploration into accreditation possibilities important. Following the Dallas II meeting, SOPHE and AAHE established the National Implementation Task Force for Accreditation in Health Education in 2007 to continue the momentum of the National Transition Task Force. Meanwhile, the CUP Model replaced the original Areas of Responsibility, Competencies, and Sub-competencies from the Role Delineation Project in the SABPAC approval requirements (SOPHE & AAHE, 2007). For CEPH leaders and other stakeholders, the CUP Model and the results of any future role delineation research needed to be an essential part of future accreditation discussions (Taub et al., 2009). Unifying the profession on accreditation for professional preparation required a unanimous acceptance and application of the current Areas of Responsibility, Competencies, and Sub- competencies as the basis for individual certification and health education practice.

Beginning in 2007, CEPH began to explore the possibility of accrediting baccalaureate public health programs, including those in community or public health education even when they were not administered in conjunction with a CEPH-accredited

Section I: Historical Perspectives

graduate-level program. After gathering input from various stakeholders and obtaining specific advice from a group of thought leaders in 2011, CEPH decided to move ahead with the development of accreditation criteria for standalone baccalaureate public health programs (SBPs). CEPH determined that the accreditation opportunity would be available to all baccalaureate public health programs, not only those with a concentration in public or community health education. Between 2011 and 2013, CEPH developed, vetted, and revised criteria and procedures to accredit SBPs. During this time, the National Implementation Task Force on Accreditation in Health Education continued to update and provide guidance to professional preparation programs in health education to prepare for CEPH accreditation. CEPH criteria for SBPs were adopted in June 2013, and CEPH accepted its first nine applications for SBP accreditation in February 2014. In a pilot study in 2014, two community health education programs mapped their curricula to both the public health core described in the CEPH criteria and the NCHEC Competencies. Figueroa, Birch, King and Cottrell (2015) found the content and skills to be complementary and the overlap substantial enough to ensure that specialty content in community health education would not be sacrificed in the new accreditation system. Once the accreditation process for SBPs began, the SABPAC approval process was officially phased out in 2015.

In the last decade, there have also been significant changes in accreditation of professional preparation programs for school health educators (Taub et al., 2014). Historically, the United States Department of Education and the Council for Higher Education Accreditation have recognized two organizations as professional accrediting bodies for teacher preparation: The National Council for Accreditation of Teacher Education (NCATE) and the Teacher Education Accreditation Council (TEAC). As of July 1, 2013, NCATE and TEAC consolidated to become the Council for the Accreditation of Educator Preparation (TEAC, 2014; CAEP, 2015). The creation of CAEP provided an opportunity to create a unified accreditation system that strengthens the performance standards of teacher education candidates, raises the stature of the teaching profession, and improves the standards for the evidence that supports claims of quality (Taub et al 2014).

Moving Forward: Continued Growth and Change

In addition to creating advanced-level certification and achieving NCCA accreditation for the CHES and MCHES certification programs, and as noted in Figure 1.1, the health education profession has continued to grow and evolve since the 1970s. The United States Department of Labor (USDOL) recognized "health educator" as a distinct standard occupational classification in 2000 (Office of Management and Budget, 2000) and predicted the occupation to grow faster than other occupations (USDOL, 2014). Employers have increasingly included CHES/MCHES "preferred" or "required" in job descriptions (Cottrell et al., 2012). Efforts have been undertaken to develop a global set of Competencies for health promotion professionals (Allegrante et al., 2009; Allegrante et al., 2012), while passage of the Patient Protection and Affordable Care Act in 2010 has further catalyzed interest in the domestic role of health education specialists in disease prevention and health promotion (SOPHE, 2013). Baccalaureate and graduate programs in public health have grown significantly in recent decades, stimulating changes in accreditation and quality assurance systems affecting health education.

Section I: Historical Perspectives

Figure 1.1

Historical Timeline of Selected Milestones

	Role Delineation/ Framework Adaptations	Professional Certification	Program Accreditation and Approval
1978	Role Delineation Project began		SOPHE initiated approval process for baccalaureate programs
1984			SABPAC established
1985	Original Entry-level Competency Framework completed		
1988		NCHEC established	
1989		First Chartered CHES	
1990		First CHES Exam offered	NCHEC continuing education/professional development system established
1992	Joint Committee for Graduate Standards created		
1998	CUP initiated		AAHE began partnering with NCATE
1999	Graduate-level Competencies completed		
2001			National Task Force on Accreditation in Health Education established
2004	CUP completed		National Transition Task Force on Accreditation in Health Education established
2005			CEPH accreditation standards for baccalaureate programs of public health schools/programs created
2006	CUP model adopted		National Implementation Task Force on Accreditation in Health Education established
2007		CUP-based CHES Exam offered	SABPAC integrated CUP model into requirements
2008	HEJA initiated	CHES program accredited by NCCA	
2009	HEJA completed		
2010	HEJA model adopted	HEJA-based MCHES EDO initiated	
2011		MCHES EDO completed First MCHES Exam offered	
2012		HEJA-based CHES Exam offered	
2013	HESPA initiated	CHES program is re-accredited and MCHES program accredited	• CEPH accreditation standards for standalone baccalaureate programs in public health created
2014	HESPA completed		• NCATE & TEAC unified to become CAEP • AAHE sunset
2015	HESPA model adopted		SABPAC sunset

Helen P. Cleary

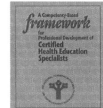
1985

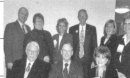
CUP Key Leaders

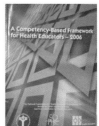
2006

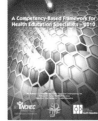
2010

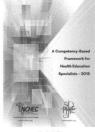
2015

Section II: HESPA 2015 Process and Outcomes

The HESPA 2015 was conducted to validate the contemporary practice of entry- and advanced-level health education specialists. The findings will be used to develop updated examinations for Certified Health Education Specialists (CHES) and Master Certified Health Education Specialists (MCHES), as well as to report validated changes in health education practice since the HEJA 2010 study and inform professional preparation and continuing education initiatives. This study was initiated in 2013 to meet accreditation standards of the National Commission for Certifying Agencies (NCCA), which requires a regular revalidation of the Competencies upon which the credential is based.

Practice analysis experts from Professional Examination Services (ProExam) oversaw the conduct of the study. ProExam adhered to the highest credentialing industry standards, using guidelines consistent with best practices as found in *The Standards for Educational and Psychological Testing* (American Educational Research Association, American Psychological Association, and National Council on Measurement in Education, 2014) and *Guidelines for the Development, Use, and Evaluation of Licensure and Certification Programs* (Professional Examination Service, 1995). These guidelines consistently have emphasized the importance of ensuring the relevance of a certification program's examination content. ProExam's work on this project was informed by practice analysis updates found in works published by Hambleton and Rogers (1986), Raymond (2002), and the NCCA (2005).

The HESPA 2015 study was guided by the principle that "health education is a single profession, with common roles and responsibilities" (Allegrante et al., 2004, p. 676). The processes used in this study were built on the work of two previous research studies in this field, HEJA 2010 (Doyle et al., 2012) and CUP (Gilmore et al., 2005).

HESPA 2015 Participants

Under the direction of ProExam, the 2015 Health Education Specialist Practice Analysis Steering Committee (HESPA 2015-SC) and the 2015 Health Education Specialist Practice Analysis Task Force (HESPA 2015-TF) led the HESPA 2015 study. The HESPA 2015-SC consisted of the chief staff officers from each sponsoring organization (i.e., NCHEC and SOPHE), the task force chair of HEJA 2010, and the two HESPA 2015-TF co-chairs appointed by NCHEC and SOPHE. The HESPA 2015-SC and ProExam employees created a *call to the profession* to assist with the study that generated a pool of more than 460 volunteer nominees. From the pool of volunteers, the HESPA 2015-SC selected 10 individuals to serve with the two HESPA 2015-TF co-chairs on the HESPA 2015-TF. The HESPA 2015-SC selected an additional 56 volunteers from this pool to serve in the *instrument development* phase of the study as subject matter experts (n=11), independent reviewers (n=20), and survey pilot participants (n=25). The HESPA 2015-TF members and the other 55 volunteers involved in creating the survey instrument represented a diversity of health education work settings, experience levels, educational backgrounds, demographic groups, and geographic settings.

The remaining participants consisted of volunteers who responded to the survey (i.e., survey participants). Two primary goals guided the recruitment of survey participants to: (a) involve as many health education specialists as possible and (b) achieve representation from all work settings, education levels, years of experience, and health education certification statuses. Because there exists no single data source for the entire group of practicing health education specialists, multiple approaches were used to invite as many health education specialists as possible to participate. The entire population of CHES and MCHES certified individuals (N=10,644), who previously granted NCHEC permission to release contact information for surveys and had e-mail addresses in the NCHEC database, was invited

Section II: HESPA 2015 Process and Outcomes

to participate. In addition, a number of strategies were employed to recruit noncertified health education specialists to participate.

First, NCHEC and SOPHE staff members identified 575 contacts at health education organizations, including member organizations of the Coalition of National Health Education Organization (CNHEO) and national and state affiliates of major health education associations responsible for electronic mailing lists. Each of these 575 contacts received an e-mail and/or personal telephone call to request organizational assistance in publicizing the study and to provide an invitation and link to the online survey registration form for their members. The identified groups participated in various capacities in advertising the study, including e-mailing information to their members and posting announcements on their Web sites.

Second, NCHEC and SOPHE staff members created Internet banners hyperlinked to the survey instrument to advertise the study on their Web sites and hyperlinked images to use as part of their e-mail signatures. The staff members of both organizations also collaborated on a special social media hash tag: #HESPA2014. NCHEC and SOPHE employed this hash tag for survey announcements posted via Twitter and Facebook. Finally, the staffs generated a HESPA Quick Response (QR) code to allow the survey registration site to be accessed via a handheld device. Staff members encouraged survey participation continually through announcements at various conferences throughout the entire survey period.

A total of 707 noncertified volunteers signed up to participate in the survey as a result of these outreach efforts. An additional 305 NCHEC certified individuals (i.e., CHES or MCHES) signed up online with e-mail addresses different from those already included in the NCHEC database. ProExam sent a total of 11,351 invitations to participate in the survey to health education specialists via e-mail. Of that number, 338 invitations were undeliverable because of invalid e-mail addresses. Another 142 invitations were declined by recipients who no longer considered themselves practicing health education specialists. Of the resulting 10,871 practicing health education specialists invited to participate, 3,152 completed the survey, resulting in a response rate of 29.0%. The health education specialists who responded represented all 50 states, the District of Columbia, and Puerto Rico, as well as a wide array of work settings (e.g., community, school, government, college/university, health care, business/industry, and academia).

HESPA 2015 Procedures

The HESPA 2015 study spanned 18 months from February 2013 to August 2014. During this period, those who conducted the study selected volunteers as previously described, developed survey instruments, and collected, analyzed, and interpreted data. The entire process consisted of the following steps (see Figure 2.1):

1. *Preliminary planning:* Preliminary plans created by the HESPA 2015-SC (February–April 2013)
2. *Volunteer selection:* Selection of the HESPA 2015-TF and other health education specialists who contributed to the development of two instruments (April–May 2013)
3. *Telephone interviews:* Preliminary telephone interviews with 11 leaders of the profession (June 2013)
4. *Task Force meeting #1:* Preliminary work by the HESPA 2015-TF to update the description of health education practice through a face-to-face meeting and follow-up activities (July–August 2013

Section II: HESPA 2015 Process and Outcomes

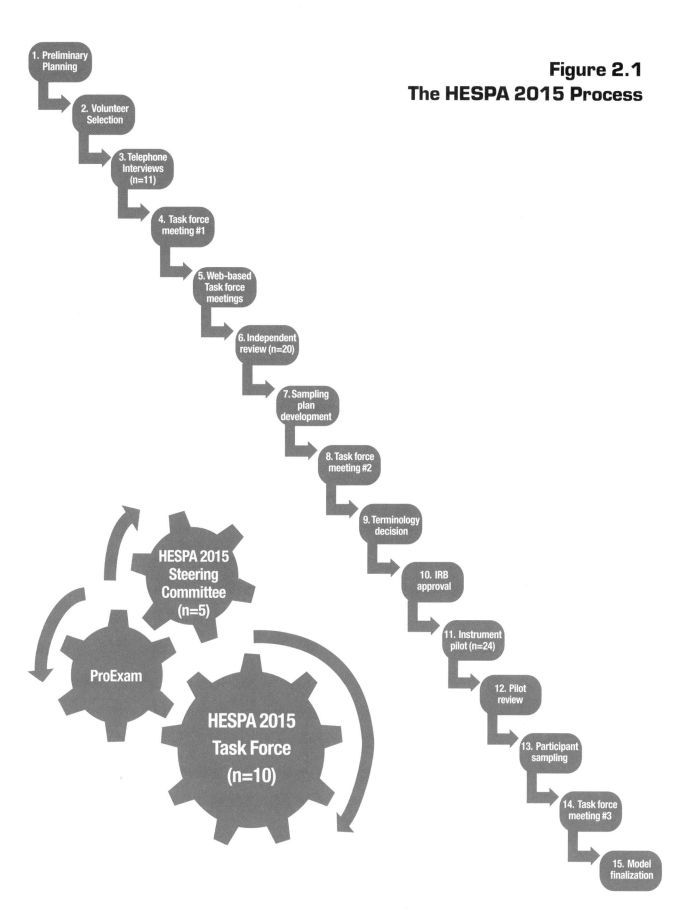

Figure 2.1
The HESPA 2015 Process

Section II: HESPA 2015 Process and Outcomes

5. *Web based Task Force meetings:* Review and further refinement of the framework by the HESPA 2015-TF via a series of five conference call meetings (September–October 2013)

6. *Independent review:* An independent review of the refined framework by 20 health education specialists representing diverse work settings (October–November 2013)

7. *Sampling plan development:* Development of a sampling plan for the validation survey by ProExam and outreach to the profession for volunteer survey participants by HESPA 2015-SC and HESPA 2015-TF members (November 2013–April 2014)

8. *Task Force meeting #2:* A face-to-face meeting of the HESPA 2015-TF to review and reconcile the independent review results, create a pre-survey iteration of the framework, and confirm survey rating scales (November 2013)

9. *Terminology decision:* Data collection initiative to obtain feedback from HESPA 2015-TF, telephone interview panel, independent review panel, the NCHEC Board of Commissioners, and the SOPHE Board of Trustees on whether or not the term health education/promotion should replace the term health education throughout the framework (December 2013)

10. *Institutional Review Board approval:* Approval of the study by the Institutional Review Board of Baylor University (January 2014)

11. *Instrument pilot:* Pilot testing of the online survey instrument for comprehensiveness, clarity, and technical ease of use by 24 health education specialists (January 2014)

12. *Pilot review:* HESPA 2015-SC subcommittee review and reconciliation of the survey instrument based upon pilot test findings (February 2014)

13. *Participant sampling:* E-mail invitations to participate in the survey sent to a valid sample of 10,871 health education specialists followed by periodic reminders sent throughout a nine week completion window, resulting in 3,152 responses and a 29.0% response rate (February–April 2014)

14. *Task Force meeting #3:* HESPA 2015-TF face-to-face meeting to review the survey results and develop recommendations to the HESPA 2015-SC (May 2014)

15. *Model finalization:* HESPA 2015-SC and ProExam employees review of the HESPA 2015-TF recommendations and finalize the HESPA Model (June–July 2014)

Conceptual Framework for Instrument Development.

As illustrated in Figure 2.1, the HESPA 2015-TF played a critical role throughout the practice analysis. The HESPA 2015-TF's work began with a review of the HEJA 2010 framework and knowledge list. From there, the HESPA 2015-TF reviewed the information that ProExam employees received after interviewing the 11 subject matter experts. Those interviews focused on changes in the health education profession since the last job analysis, items missing from the HEJA 2010 framework, and knowledge and skills required for health education specialists to be competent practitioners in the years ahead. After reviewing the HEJA 2010 framework and the interviews, the HESPA 2015-TF created the first iteration of the HESPA 2015 Model. Once the HESPA 2015-TF created the initial HESPA 2015 Model, the HESPA 2015-TF tasked 20 independent reviewers

Section II: HESPA 2015 Process and Outcomes

to review and provide feedback on the initial Model. Finally, the HESPA 2015-TF used that feedback to shape the piloted HESPA 2015 Model. Throughout the model development process, ProExam practice analysis experts, recommendations from practicing health education specialists, and emerging professional trends evident in the HEJA 2010 Model and the *Report of the 2011 Joint Committee on Health Education and Promotion Terminology* (Joint Committee on Health Education and Promotion Terminology, 2012) guided the HESPA 2015-TF.

In the early stages of updating the Areas of Responsibility, Competencies, and Sub-competencies for use in the study, HESPA 2015-TF members discussed the types and depth of knowledge that health education specialists needed to possess to effectively perform a specific Competency or Sub-competency. This topic arose most frequently during discussions regarding current practice and the long-range use of study outcomes to shape professional preparation and development efforts. Like the HEJA 2010-TF members before them, HESPA 2015-TF members agreed that a Competency-based approach to professional preparation, credentialing, and development was essential.

Also as with HEJA 2010, the HESPA 2015-TF members recognized the utility of identifying relevant knowledge items to be included in professional preparation and continuing education programs. For this reason, the HESPA 2015-TF members decided to collect survey data to again verify knowledge items. The HESPA 2015-TF members used similar procedures as used in the HEJA 2010 study to compose the 132 knowledge items for the HESPA 2015 survey. Therefore, the piloted instrument included 273 Sub-competency statements and 132 knowledge statements.

Survey Instrument. As previously indicated, a group of 25 health education specialists were asked to pilot test the online survey instrument. Of that number, 24 (96%) completed the pilot test. This pilot test revealed that respondents were taking a long time to complete the instrument. Although the HESPA 2015-TF considered creating several versions of survey instrument, each containing a subset of Sub-competency elements to reduce survey fatigue, they ultimately decided to retain all Sub-competencies in one version of the survey. The HESPA 2015-TF made this decision out of concern that random routing within the Sub-competency areas may direct respondents to areas in which they had little experience. Although multiple survey versions might have contributed to higher completion rates and less survey fatigue, the HESPA 2015-TF concluded the advantages of retaining all Sub-competencies in one version of the survey outweighed the possible disadvantages. Ultimately, the HESPA 2015-TF decided to create two versions of the instrument: one version focused on Sub-competencies and one version focused on knowledge items. In this way, conceptually-related items (i.e., Sub-competencies or knowledge) could be rated within a single instrument by a subset of respondents.

The HESPA 2015-TF devoted much time to a discussion of the rating scales to be used in the survey. The HESPA 2015-TF considered various Likert-type rating scales and ultimately decided to use the same rating scales employed in the CUP and the HEJA 2010 studies to permit comparisons of the HESPA 2015 findings with those in the previous two studies. Participants who completed the Sub-competency version instrument rated each Sub-competency in terms of:
- Frequency of practice within the past 12 months: *Not at all, occasionally (less than once a month), frequently (at least once each month, very frequently (at least once each week)*

Section II: HESPA 2015 Process and Outcomes

- Importance of the Sub-competency to the participant's work: *Not important, minimally important, moderately important, highly important*

The participants rated the Areas of Responsibility using two scales designed to gather information on the percentage of work time that they spent performing the activities in each Area as well as the importance of the Area.
- What percentage of your work time as a health education specialist was spent in each Area of Responsibility over the past 12 months?
- Importance of the Sub-competency to the participant's work: *Not important, minimally important, moderately important, highly important*

The HESPA 2015-TF also discussed potential rating scales for the knowledge statements, including the scale used in HEJA 2010 to evaluate the cognitive level at which respondents used the knowledge items. Ultimately, the HESPA 2015-TF adopted the frequency scale used to rate the Sub-competencies to rate the statements on the knowledge version of the survey instrument.
- Frequency of practice within the past 12 months: *Not at all, occasionally (less than once a month), frequently (at least once each month, very frequently (at least once each week)*

Both the Sub-competency and the knowledge versions of the survey instruments included 17 demographic and professional questions to elicit information on key characteristics of respondents. Key characteristics included education and experience levels, work setting, type of work performed, professional credentials, organizational memberships, and race/ethnicity.

The Sub-competency version instrument included a total of 291 items (one screening question, 273 Sub-competencies organized into 36 Competencies and framed within Seven Areas of Responsibility, and 17 demographic and professional questions), while the knowledge version instrument included 150 items (one screening question, 132 knowledge items, and 17 demographic and professional questions).

Analysis and Outcomes

ProExam employees compiled survey responses, performed data reduction and analysis, and guided the HESPA 2015-TF in the interpretation of the results. As a part of this work, ProExam employees: (a) developed demographic profiles of participants (group percentages) based on certification status (i.e., CHES or MCHES vs. non-CHES or non-MCHES), educational degrees earned, years of experience, and work setting and (b) developed subgroup analyses based upon work settings, years of experience, certification status, and education levels. All analyses were performed using Statistical Package for the Social Sciences (SPSS) v22.0.

Demographics. The 3,152 survey participants represented all 50 states, the District of Columbia, and Puerto Rico, while 49 respondents indicated they were working outside of the United States. The largest percentages of participants were from California (8.7%, n=271), Georgia (6.0%, n=186), and Texas (5.7%, n=178). A majority of the participants identified as female (89.4%, n=2,779), White/Caucasian (69.4%, n=2,142), and less than 46 years old (74.7%, n=2,312). A majority also indicated that they worked full-time (65.7%, n=2,054), and completed a master's degree as their highest level of education (60.1%, n=1,856) (see Table 2.1).

Section II: HESPA 2015 Process and Outcomes

Table 2.1

Demographic Data of Survey Participants (N=3,152)

Characteristic	n*	%
Gender		
Female	2779	89.4
Male	294	9.5
Prefer not to answer	36	1.2
Race/Ethnicity		
American Indian or Alaskan Native	24	0.8
Asian	131	4.2
Black or African American	392	12.7
Hispanic or Latino/Latina	204	6.6
White or Caucasian	2142	69.4
More than one racial or ethnic background	73	2.4
Other	31	1.0
Prefer not to answer	90	2.9
Age		
25 years and under	390	12.6
26–35 years	1262	40.8
36–45 years	660	21.3
46–55 years	376	12.1
56–65 years	308	9.9
66–75 years	47	1.5
76 years and older	3	0.1
Prefer not to answer	50	1.6
Employment status		
Full-time	2054	65.7
Part-time	565	18.1
Not currently working as a Health Education Specialist	506	16.2
Education (highest level of degree earned)		
Baccalaureate degree	794	25.8
Master's degree	1856	60.1
Health Education Specialist degree	3	0.1
Doctorate	431	14.0

*Not all totals add up to N=3,152 because of missing data.

Section II: HESPA 2015 Process and Outcomes

A majority of participants (80.0%, n=2,523) held the CHES credential, while about one-seventh of the participants held the MCHES credential (13.7%, n=432). Eighty-seven participants (2.8%) indicated they held the Certified in Public Health (CPH) credential, and another 101 (3.2%) participants held the Child Passenger Safety credential. A majority of participants (58.9%, n=1,825) had worked as a health education specialist for five or more years, while the mean number of years of service as a health education specialist was 8.9 years. Just about two-thirds of the participants (66.7%, n=2,015) indicated they had worked in their current position between one and four years, and less than one-fifth (17.1%, n=532) indicated that they had been responsible for supervising other health education specialists. When asked about membership in professional associations, 847 (26.9%) indicated they were members of SOPHE, 636 (20.2%) were members of the American Public Health Association (APHA), and 597 (18.9%) indicated they were members of a local, state, and regional organizations. The greatest number of participants (31.1%, n=980) indicated that they did not belong to any professional association (see Table 2.2).

Section II: HESPA 2015 Process and Outcomes

Table 2.2

Professional Data of Survey Participants (N=3,152)

Characteristic	n*	%
NCHEC certification status		
CHES	2523	80.0
MCHES	432	13.7
Never held CHES or MCHES	179	5.7
Lapsed CHES or MCHES	18	0.6
Other certifications dealing with health education/promotion		
Certified in Public Health (CPH)	87	2.8
Certified Diabetes Educator (CDE)	13	0.4
Certified Asthma Educator	10	0.3
Certified Prevention Professional (CPP)	14	0.4
Certified Prevention Specialist (CPS)	24	0.8
Child Passenger Safety	101	3.2
Years experience as a health education specialist		
Less than 5 years	1275	41.1
5 or more years	25	58.9
Years in current position		
1 year or less	1057	35.0
2 to 4 years	958	31.7
5 to 7 years	413	13.7
8 to 10 years	250	8.3
11 to 15 years	169	5.6
16 years or more	173	5.7
Supervise other health education specialists		
Yes	532	17.1
No	2585	82.9
If yes, number supervised		
1 to 5	390	76.0
6 to 10	72	14.0
11 to 15	23	4.5
16 to 20	15	2.9
20+	13	2.5

Section II: HESPA 2015 Process and Outcomes

Table 2.2
Professional Data of Survey Participants (N=3,152)

Characteristic	n*	%
Membership in health education professional associations		
Society for Public Health Education (SOPHE)	847	26.9
American Public Health Association – Public Health Education and Health Promotion Section (APHA-PHEHP)	585	18.6
American Public Health Association – School Health Education and Services Section (APHA-SHES)	51	1.6
American College Health Association (ACHA)	128	4.1
American School Health Association (ASHA)	103	3.3
Directors of Health Promotion and Education (DHPE)	34	1.1
Eta Sigma Gamma (ESG)	282	8.9
American Academy of Health Behavior (AAHB)	12	0.4
American College of Sports Medicine (ACSM)	73	2.3
International Union for Health Promotion and Education (IUHPE)	22	0.7
National Public Health Information Coalition (NPHIC)	13	0.4
Society of Health and Physical Educators (SHAPE America)/American Association or Health, Physical Education, Recreation and Dance	111	3.5
Society of State Leaders of Health and Physical Education	8	0.3
Local, state, or regional affiliate of a national organization	597	18.9
None of these	980	31.1
Other	369	11.7

*Not all totals add up to N=3,152 because of missing data.

Of the 3,152 participants, 3,117 (98.9%) indicated their primary work setting (see Table 2.3). The greatest percentage of participants identified their work setting as the government (20.8%, n=650), followed by health care (19.0%, n=592), academia (16.4%, n=511), community (15.7%, n=490), business/worksite (10.7%, n=334), college health (6.8%, n=213), other (6.6%, n=203), and school health (4.0%, n=124) settings. The seven major categories of work settings reflect the range of settings where contemporary health education specialists work.

Section II: HESPA 2015 Process and Outcomes

Table 2.3
Work Settings of Survey Participants (N=3,117)

	n	%
Community	**490**	**15.7%**
Health planning agency	17	0.5%
Voluntary health agency	26	0.8%
Nonprofit health education center	89	2.9%
Nonprofit health organization	337	10.8%
Other community	21	0.7%
Health Care	**592**	**19.0%**
Hospital	341	10.9%
Non-hospital health care facility	121	3.9%
Health plan	71	2.3%
Managed care organization	49	1.6%
Other health care	10	0.3%
Government	**650**	**20.8%**
Municipal, county, or district department or agency	303	9.7%
State department or agency	218	7.0%
Federal department or agency	128	4.1%
Other government	1	0.0%
School Health	**124**	**4.0%**
Pre-K, elementary and/or secondary school	73	2.3%
School district	42	1.3%
State education department	8	0.3%
Other school health	1	0.0%
Business/Worksite	**334**	**10.7%**
Business or industry	87	2.8%
Worksite	136	4.4%
Health insurance	67	2.1%
For profit contracting agency	39	1.3%
Organized labor	4	0.1%
Other business/worksite	1	0.0%
Academia	**511**	**16.4%**
Academia (college or university)	511	16.4%
College Health	**213**	**6.8%**
University or college health services	213	6.8%
Other	**203**	**6.6%**
Self employed	92	3.0%
Professional association	18	0.6%
Military	24	0.8%
Intergovernmental organizations	10	0.3%
International/NGO	16	0.5%
Other	31	1.0%
Unemployed	12	0.4%
Total	3117	100.0%

Section II: HESPA 2015 Process and Outcomes

Generic Sub-competencies. Replicating a process used in prior studies (Doyle et al., 2012; Gilmore, et al., 2005), ProExam employees calculated composite scores for each Sub-competency using the formula: *(frequency – 1) + importance*. The composite score generated for each Sub-competency represented a stronger weighting for the *importance* of a Sub-competency to the job in relation to the frequency at which health education specialists practiced. This method of weighting resulted in the lowest scores for Sub-competencies which participants deemed both unimportant and infrequently performed as indicated by a composite score of less than 3.0.

The HESPA 2015-TF defined generic Sub-competencies as those Sub-competencies performed by health education specialists *regardless* of practice setting. Guidelines for the validation of generic Sub-competencies were based on subgroup analyses of the composite scores by work setting, similar to those methods employed in the CUP and HEJA 2010 Models. To be identified as generic Sub-competency, the HESPA 2015-TF decided that Sub-competencies had to have a composite score of at least 3.0 (on a 7-point scale) in five of the seven practice settings (excluding the "other" category). All 273 Sub-competencies met the 3.0 mean composite score threshold and were retained in the framework.

Entry- and Advanced-level Sub-competencies. One important goal of the HESPA 2015 study was to develop a framework to describe the practice of the health education profession. To explore if the hierarchical structure validated through the CUP and HEJA 2010 Models was still a useful way to delineate practice, ProExam employees ran subgroup analyses on the composite score ratings along a variety of dimensions. Repeated pairwise comparisons between the composite scores from subgroups were conducted for each Sub-competency using two sided tests and assuming equal variances with a significance level 0.05. Given the large number of pairwise comparisons conducted, ProExam employees used the Bonferroni correction to reduce the possibility of Type I error.

ProExam employees examined both statistical and substantive differences in Sub-competency mean composite scores to determine if there were differences in the salience of the Sub-competencies for health education specialists who varied on 90 dimensions, such as years of experience and highest degree earned. The American Psychological Association (APA) Board of Scientific Affairs has supported the reliance on a combination of the statistical significance and the magnitude of observed results as a basis to draw an informed inference about those results (Wilkinson & Task Force for Statistical Inference, 1999). For example, in some cases a large number of responses presented with a small standard deviation in the responses. These instances represented statistical differences with very small magnitudes. In such cases, the small magnitude of the differences indicated that subgroups have essentially similar patterns of responses. In these cases, relying on purely significant differences was not sufficient to determine the real differences between groups.

The first subgroup comparison arranged respondents with up to five years of experience in one subgroup and respondents with five or more years of experience in the other subgroup. This comparison was used in both the CUP and HEJA 2010 Models to make the preliminary categorization of Sub-competencies into entry- and advanced-levels. The results of this analysis did not yield clear distinctions for classifying Sub-competencies into levels of practice. Differences were small in magnitude. Only five of the 273 Sub-competencies had differences in composite scores equal to 0.5 (on a 7-point scale), and only 12 Sub-competencies had differences equal to 0.4. In this respect, the data analyses in the current study did not replicate the findings of CUP and HEJA 2010 studies in which the ratings of respondents with less than five years of

Section II: HESPA 2015 Process and Outcomes

experience differed significantly from the ratings of those with five or more years of experience. HESPA subgroup analyses based on five years of experience did not provide clear guidance for categorizing Sub-competencies as entry- or advanced-level. This change might reflect changes in the profession related to the assumption of different types or greater amounts of responsibility at an earlier point in the health education specialists' professional development.

This shift might also reflect an increase in outreach to survey respondents from a wider range of organizations and with less clear patterns of practice. The initial analyses did not permit using five years of experience as the primary determinant for classifying entry- and advanced-level Sub-competencies. Therefore, the ProExam employees conducted a variety of other subgroup analyses to explore patterns in ratings that might be linked to entry- and advanced-level practice. The additional subgroup analyses were conducted by:
- the highest degree earned in a health education major,
- a combinations of experience and education (baccalaureate with less than 5 years of experience, baccalaureate with 5 or more years, master's with less than 5 years, master's with 5 or more years, doctorate with less than 5 years, doctorate with 5 or more years), and
- certification status (CHES or MCHES or non-certified).

In addition, there was virtually no substantive or statistically significant difference between the two groups of respondents with doctoral degrees (i.e., those with up to 5 years of experience and those with 5 or more years of experience). Therefore the two respondent groups with doctoral degrees were merged for all future analyses.

All of these subgroups were selected by ProExam employees in consultation with the HESPA 2015-SC for further analysis based on the patterns of practice which survey ratings revealed may have differed between the subgroups identified. For example, the highest level of education attained in a health education major was used in the CUP and HEJA 2010 Models to distinguish between advanced 1- and advanced 2-level Sub-competencies and explore patterns of ratings in the current study as well. In the HESPA 2015 study, combinations of education, certification status, and experience levels were used to compare respondents with lower terminal degrees but who had more experience to respondents with higher terminal degrees at the beginning of their careers. These new data on certification have provided another way to examine practice and have provided results that may aid NCHEC in the development of test content for the two credentialing examinations.

During its third face-to-face third meeting, the HESPA 2015-TF made recommendations regarding the allocation of Sub-competencies to the entry-, advanced 1-, and advanced 2-levels of practice based on the results of the repeated pairwise comparisons between the composite scores from subgroups for each Sub-competency. Due to time constraints and requests from members of the HESPA 2015-TF for additional information regarding the survey ratings, this task could not be completed during the meeting. One such request questioned the efficacy of the cut point that ProExam implemented for the years of experience: less than five years versus five or more years. The HESPA 2015-TF referred further consideration of the criteria for categorizing Sub-competencies into levels to the HESPA 2015-SC for further analysis. After the meeting, the HESPA 2015-SC requested that ProExam undertake additional data analyses to explore the efficacy of different cut points.

Refinement and Finalization of the Framework. Upon the request of HESPA 2015-SC, ProExam employees conducted additional data analyses.

Section II: HESPA 2015 Process and Outcomes

First, ProExam employees performed a Rasch analysis using Facets to transform the ordinal composite scores into logit values on an interval scale. Through this conversion process, 77 participants were identified as having provided responses to the survey instrument questions that were anomalous and were, in statistical terms, "ill fitting to the model." Data for all 77 cases were eliminated from subsequent analyses. All analyses were rerun after eliminating the 77 cases. There were no substantive changes in the findings. Next, using the Sub-competency logit values, ProExam employees conducted a discriminant analysis to identify the number of years of experience that best differentiated entry- from advanced-level practice. ProExam employees ran the analysis using cut points of 2, 3, 4, 5, 6, 7, and 8 years of experience.

After the second analysis of the data, the HESPA 2015-SC met with ProExam employees to review the results. Based upon this analysis, the HESPA 2015-SC found the data did not support a change in the cut point from five years to any other cut point. The HESPA 2015-SC then created a series of data driven rules that took into consideration the statistically significant differences between the various subgroups based on education and years of experience, as well as the magnitude of the differences found to determine the placement of Sub-competencies into the entry-, advanced 1-, or advanced 2-levels of practice.

After placing all 273 Sub-competencies into levels, the HESPA 2015-SC examined the possibility of combining like Sub-competencies. For the purposes of this research, several Sub-competencies that were essentially identical except for the leading action verb or the object of the action were included in the survey as separate line items. The items were included in the survey separately to test the hypothesis that health education specialists at different levels of professional development might use the Sub-competencies differently. Based on the nature of the activity, it was expected that the Sub-competencies might represent either entry- or advanced-levels of practice. The following pairs of Sub-competencies represent examples of parallel Sub-competencies surveyed separately: (a) *Identify factors that influence health behaviors* and *Analyze factors that influence health behaviors* and (b) *Address diversity within priority populations in selecting strategies/interventions* and *Address diversity within priority populations in designing strategies/interventions*.

The findings ultimately supported combining 15 pairs of such parallel Sub-competencies, which had already been placed at the same level of practice. Therefore, the parallel Sub-competencies in these 15 cases were combined. The Sub-competencies ultimately were presented, for example, as: (a) *Identify and analyze factors that influence health behaviors* and (b) *Address diversity within priority populations in selecting and/or designing strategies/interventions*. This review and categorization process by the HESPA 2015-SC reduced the number of Sub-competencies in the framework from 273 to 258.

After the HESPA 2015-SC completed its review, the Model was forwarded to the HESPA 2015-TF via e-mail for review and comment. The HESPA 2015-SC members received several comments from the HESPA 2015-TF, yet none of the comments was expressed by a majority of the members. Therefore, no additional changes were made to the HESPA 2015 Model.

The Validated Model. Through the HESPA 2015 process, the Model of the practice of health education has been updated, refined, and validated. The HESPA 2015 Model now consists of 258 Sub-competencies organized into 36 Competencies within the Seven Areas of Responsibility:

Section II: HESPA 2015 Process and Outcomes

> **Seven Areas of Responsibility of Health Education Specialists**
>
> I. Assess Needs, Resources, and Capacity for Health Education/Promotion
> II. Plan Health Education/Promotion
> III. Implement Health Education/Promotion
> IV. Conduct Evaluation and Research Related to Health Education/Promotion
> V. Administer and Manage Health Education/Promotion
> VI. Serve as a Health Education/Promotion Resource Person
> VII. Communicate, Promote, and Advocate for Health, Health Education/Promotion, and the Profession

The results of the HESPA 2015 study reverified the three distinct levels of practice established in the CUP and HEJA 2010 Models, i.e., the entry-, advanced 1-, and advanced 2-levels. In addition to the Areas of Responsibilities and Competencies, the HESPA 2015 study also identified 258 Sub-competencies. Those validated at the entry-level are required for health education specialists near the beginning of their professional development. Additional Sub-competencies have been validated only for more experienced health education specialists, although more experienced practitioners are still expected to be competent in the entry-level Sub-competencies. Specific numbers of Competencies and Sub-competencies for each Area of Responsibility are listed below. Section III provides more details about the HESPA Model.

Area of Responsibility I: 7 Competencies – 33 Sub-competencies
- 30 entry-level
- 3 advanced 1-level
- 0 advanced 2-level

Area of Responsibility II: 5 Competencies – 34 Sub-competencies
- 28 entry-level
- 6 advanced 1-level
- 0 advanced 2-level

Area of Responsibility III: 4 Competencies – 29 Sub-competencies
- 21 entry-level
- 8 advanced 1-level
- 0 advanced 2-level

Area of Responsibility IV: 7 Competencies – 57 Sub-competencies
- 9 entry-level
- 10 advanced 1-level
- 38 advanced 2-level

Section II: HESPA 2015 Process and Outcomes

Area of Responsibility V: 6 Competencies – 51 Sub-competencies
- 18 entry-level
- 33 advanced 1-level
- 0 advanced 2-level

Area of Responsibility VI: 3 Competencies – 16 Sub-competencies
- 5 entry-level
- 11 advanced 1-level
- 0 advanced 2-level

Area of Responsibility VII: 4 Competencies – 38 Sub-competencies
- 30 entry-level
- 5 advanced 1-level
- 3 advanced 2-level

Verified Knowledge Items. A newly generated list of 131 verified knowledge items organized into 10 conceptually related topic areas emerged from this study. The conceptually related areas include: Health Education Profession; Theories, Techniques; Ethics; Capacity, Community Building; Systems; Research, Evaluation, Data Collection; Management, Budget, Administration, Human Resources; Communication; Advocacy; and Other. As noted earlier, participants rated the knowledge items based on how frequently they used the knowledge in their job as a health education specialist during the previous 12 months. To be verified, the knowledge items had to be used at a level of frequency greater than *Never* by at least 50% of all health education specialists. Five cases did not meet this threshold. In four instances, where fewer than 50% of respondents used the knowledge, if at least one work setting used the knowledge on a level of at least *Occasionally*, the knowledge area was retained in the list of verified terms. The four knowledge areas used by fewer than 50% of all respondents but used at least *Occasionally* in at least one major work setting were: *School health education, professional preparation and licensure* (school health setting); *Public health, non-US systems* (academia); *Fundraising, principles and methods, legal issues* (community); and *Media advocacy* (community). Lobbying was the only knowledge item eliminated after not being verified. Section VI includes a list of these knowledge items and an overview of recommendations for their use.

Discussion

Validated Areas of Responsibilities, Competencies, and Sub-competencies. The HESPA 2015 Model represents the fourth time the health education profession has validated the Areas of Responsibility, Competencies, and Sub-competencies. This iteration revealed that the number of Areas of Responsibility remained the same, while the number of Competencies and Sub-competencies increased. Although such an expansion may signify an expanded role of the health education specialist, the expansion more likely has occurred because of the new strategies and technologies that are available and the greater delineation within the role.

In this iteration of the Areas of Responsibility, Competencies, and Sub-competencies, the biggest fluctuations in the total number Sub-competencies from HEJA 2010 to HESPA 2015 have occurred in

Section II: HESPA 2015 Process and Outcomes

two areas: *Area of Responsibility IV: Conduct Evaluation and Research Related to Health Education/Promotion* and *Area of Responsibility V: Administer and Manage Health Education/Promotion*. The number of Sub-competencies in *Area of Responsibility IV* increased from 34 in the HEJA 2010 Model to 57 in HESPA 2015 Model. Similarly, the number of Sub-competencies in *Area of Responsibility V* increased from 31 in the HEJA 2010 Model to 51 in the HESPA 2015 Model. The expansion might best be explained by the maturity of the profession. Health education specialists may now be able to better distinguish between the skills and knowledge needed in these more advanced roles.

The greatest percentage of entry-level Sub-competencies has been validated in *Area of Responsibility I: Assess Needs, Resources, and Capacity for Health Education/Promotion* (90.9% validated at entry-level). This validation was followed by *Area of Responsibility II: Plan Health Education/Promotion* (82.4% validated at entry-level); *Area of Responsibility VII: Communicate, Promote, and Advocate for Health, Health Education/Promotion and the Profession* (78.9% validated at entry-level); *Area of Responsibility III: Implement Health Education/Promotion* (72.4% validated at entry-level); *Area of Responsibility V: Administer and Manage Health Education/Promotion* (35.3% validated at entry-level); *Area of Responsibility VI: Serve as a Health Education/Promotion Resource Person* (31.3% validated at entry-level); and *Area of Responsibility IV: Conduct Evaluation and Research Related to Health Education/Promotion* (15.8% validated at entry-level). The greatest percentage of advanced-level Sub-competencies has been validated in *Area of Responsibility IV: Conduct Evaluation and Research Related to Health Education/Promotion* (84.2% validated at advanced-level), followed by *Area of Responsibility VI: Serve as a Health Education/Promotion Resource Person* (68.7% validated at advanced-level), as well as *Area of Responsibility V: Administer and Manage Health Education/Promotion* (64.7% validated at advanced-level). These validations seem appropriate given that many advanced 2-level health education specialists are involved in research and evaluation studies. The Area with the most advanced 2-level Sub-competencies was *Area of Responsibility IV: Conduct Evaluation and Research Related to Health Education/Promotion* (66.7% validated at the advanced 2-level). The only other Area of Responsibility with advanced-2 level Sub-competencies was *Area of Responsibility VII: Communicate, Promote, and Advocate for Health, Health Education/Promotion, and the Profession* (7.9% validated at advanced 2-level).

Verified Knowledge Items. The HESPA 2015 study is the second attempt to validate knowledge items within the profession. The HEJA 2010 Model represents the first attempt (Doyle et al., 2012). The validated knowledge items provide a summary of the foundational knowledge that health education specialists should possess to perform the Seven Areas of Responsibility effectively.

As noted by those involved in the creation of the first list, the initial validated knowledge list may not have been exhaustive. This newer list also may not be exhaustive. However, this Model includes 131 terms and 18 more than the previous list. This list (see Section VI) also includes the grouping of those terms into 10 conceptually related topics whereas the previous Model presented these terms alphabetically. This new grouping offers support to health education specialists who use the list to develop curricula or exams, plan course content, or create continuing education opportunities. As the profession moves forward, this knowledge list should expand, contract, and evolve to meet the dynamic nature of the health education profession.

Section II: HESPA 2015 Process and Outcomes

Summary

The HESPA 2015 Model validates the contemporary practice of entry- and advanced-level health education specialists. The 15 steps illustrated in Figure 2.1 outline the work of 67 volunteer professionals representing a diversity of health education work settings, educational backgrounds, and experience levels within the profession. In addition to the five-member HESPA 2015-SC, these volunteers included the 10-member HESPA 2015-TF, 11 subject matter experts, 20 independent reviewers, and 24 subject matter experts who completed the pilot instrument. With support from the HESPA 2015-SC, the HESPA 2015-TF worked with the ProExam experts to complete 18 months of planning, execution, data analyses, and model development.

The HESPA 2015 Model has yielded an updated, refined, and validated framework that outlines the current practice of health education specialists at three levels: entry-, advanced 1-, and advanced 2-levels. In addition, the knowledge base supporting the work of health education specialists has been organized into a conceptual structure and verified. The final framework consists of 258 Sub-competencies organized into 36 Competencies within Seven Areas of Responsibility. Of the Sub-competencies, 141 (54.7%) have been validated at entry-level, 76 (29.5%) have been validated at the advanced 1-level, and 41 (15.9%) have been validated at the advanced 2-level. The knowledge base needed by health education specialists has been organized into 10 conceptual topic areas, and 131 knowledge topics have been validated as being used by health education specialists. More details about the HESPA 2015 Model and knowledge list, as well as recommendations for their use, are included in subsequent sections of this publication. A comparison of the HESPA 2015 Model with the CUP and HEJA 2010 Models is also provided.

Section III: The HESPA 2015 Model

The HESPA 2015 Model (see Table 3.1) contains a set of Competencies and Sub-competencies used in both the entry- and advanced-levels practice of health education specialists. These Competencies and Sub-competencies are generic across work settings and serve as the basis for professional preparation, credentialing, and professional development for all health education specialists. As with both the CUP and HEJA 2010 frameworks, it is recommended that the HESPA 2015 entry-level Competencies and Sub-competencies be addressed in undergraduate and graduate programs. Graduate programs also should incorporate the advanced 1- and advanced 2-level Competencies and Sub-competencies with doctoral programs giving specific emphasis to the advanced 2-level Competencies.

It is possible that additional setting-specific Competencies and Sub-competencies may be needed in professional preparation and development efforts for some work settings. For example, those working in health care settings may need more preparation in the culture of health care organizations; those working in community health settings may need a working knowledge of public health policy; in some business or corporate settings, the application of worksite safety regulations may be needed; and, for those preparing to teach in schools teaching methodologies may be needed.

The format used to present the Areas of Responsibility, Competencies, and Sub-competencies is the same numbering system that was developed for and used in the HEJA 2010 Model. This numbering system was retained for the HESPA 2015 Model to provide a simple and consistent approach to label and use parts of the Model. Roman numerals still will be used when referring to the Seven Areas of Responsibility when the Areas stand alone, though Arabic numbers will be used as part of the numbering system for the Areas when referring to Competencies and Sub-competencies. In this numbering system, the first number refers to the Area of Responsibility, the second number refers to the Competency within that Area, and the third number refers to the Sub-competency. For example, the three digit number 1.2.3 represents the third Sub-competency, under the second

Table 3.1

Health Education Specialist Practice Analysis 2015 Model: Overview of Areas of Responsibility and Competencies

Area of Responsibility I: Assess Needs, Resources, and Capacity for Health Education/Promotion
- 1.1 Plan assessment process for health education/promotion
- 1.2 Access existing information and data related to health
- 1.3 Collect primary data to determine needs
- 1.4 Analyze relationships among behavioral, environmental, and other factors that influence health
- 1.5 Examine factors that influence the process by which people learn
- 1.6 Examine factors that enhance or impede the process of health education/promotion
- 1.7 Determine needs for health education/promotion based on assessment findings

Section III: The HESPA 2015 Model

Area of Responsibility II: Plan Health Education/Promotion
  2.1 Involve priority populations, partners, and other stakeholders in the planning process
  2.2 Develop goals and objectives
  2.3 Select or design strategies/interventions
  2.4 Develop a plan for the delivery of health education/promotion
  2.5 Address factors that influence implementation of health education/promotion

Area of Responsibility III: Implement Health Education/Promotion
  3.1 Coordinate logistics necessary to implement plan
  3.2 Train staff members and volunteers involved in implementation of health education/promotion
  3.3 Implement health education/promotion plan
  3.4 Monitor implementation of health education/promotion

Area of Responsibility IV: Conduct Evaluation and Research Related to Health Education/Promotion
  4.1 Develop evaluation plan for health education/promotion
  4.2 Develop a research plan for health education/promotion
  4.3 Select, adapt, and/or create instruments to collect data
  4.4 Collect and manage data
  4.5 Analyze data
  4.6 Interpret results
  4.7 Apply findings

Area of Responsibility V: Administer and Manage Health Education/Promotion
  5.1 Manage financial resources for health education/promotion programs
  5.2 Manage technology resources
  5.3 Manage relationships with partners and other stakeholders
  5.4 Gain acceptance and support for health education/promotion programs
  5.5 Demonstrate leadership
  5.6 Manage human resources for health education/promotion programs

Area of Responsibility VI: Serve as a Health Education/Promotion Resource Person
  6.1 Obtain and disseminate health-related information
  6.2 Train others to use health education/promotion skills
  6.3 Provide advice and consultation on health education/promotion issues

Area of Responsibility VII: Communicate, Promote, and Advocate for Health, Health Education/Promotion, and the Profession
  7.1 Identify, develop, and deliver messages using a variety of communication strategies, methods, and techniques
  7.2 Engage in advocacy for health and health education/promotion
  7.3 Influence policy and/or systems change to promote health and health education
  7.4 Promote the health education profession

Section III: The HESPA 2015 Model

Area of Responsibility I: Assess Needs, Resources, and Capacity for Health Education/Promotion

The Role. The primary purpose of a needs, resources, and capacity assessment is to gather data and information to determine what interventions would be appropriate in a given setting. To successfully conduct a needs assessment, health education specialists must determine the purpose and scope of the assessment, collect appropriate data (i.e., primary and secondary), analyze the data, prioritize the needs, and identify the program focus. To assess the capacity of the priority population, health education specialists also must identify the available resources to address the needs and determine the extent of existing services and gaps in the provision of services (see Table 3.2).

Settings. The following text is presented to describe how assessment is used in different practice settings.

Community Setting. In a community setting, health education specialists rely on many sources of primary and secondary data to determine the needs of those in the priority population. Such data can come from health planning agencies, public health departments, census reports, data sets (e.g., Behavioral Risk Factor Surveillance Systems and Youth Risk Behavioral Surveillance Systems), and interviews with community leaders and members within the priority population. Data provide information about both real and perceived health needs. Depending on the types of needs identified, a well-planned health education program could be the way to address these needs. For example, if specific behaviors or health practices are causally linked to the incidence of major health problems, then a health program can be planned to motivate and facilitate voluntary, desirable changes in those behaviors.

School (K-12) Setting. Local, state, and national data are used to determine the scope and sequence of curricula in a school setting, as well as to identify strengths and weaknesses that aid in developing a Whole School, Whole Community, Whole Child (WSCC) model program. National and state data may be considered and utilized, but local data are essential to good curriculum planning. Information about health knowledge, attitudes, skills, and practices can be gathered directly from students and used to improve health instruction, school policies, and school environment. Information gathered from parents, administrators, and school health personnel by a "School Health Team," consisting of representatives from each of the key areas of the WSCC model, may assist in identifying potential gaps in creating a healthy school community.

Health Care Setting. In a health care setting, complaints by health professionals about a growing number of emergency room visits might lead health education specialists to survey patients' medical records to determine whether the problem is general or limited to patients with particular kinds of emergencies or situational needs (e.g., patients without adequate health insurance or with limited access to primary care physicians). An assessment of the reasons for a given trend may help to determine what services or policies could improve the situation. Health education specialists also may survey patients in a clinic to assess needs for, and interests in, educational programs offered in the clinical practice. When delivering health coaching in a clinic setting, health education specialists may assess patients' knowledge, perceptions, attitudes, and motivations regarding their current health status, as well as any potential changes the patients may be considering to improve or maintain their health. Health education specialists might accomplish this assessment by interviewing the patients and reviewing medical records of the patients.

Section III: The HESPA 2015 Model

Area of Responsibility I: Assess Needs, Resources, and Capacity for Health Education/Promotion

Business/Industry Setting. In the workplace, health education specialists might work with medical professionals and/or health insurance carriers to analyze data that can be used to identify the health needs of workers. For example, this analysis might include data about health insurance claims, predictive modeling (future risk projections), disease prevalence, absenteeism and its causes, types of accidents and severity of injuries, and compensation claims. In addition, health education specialists in this setting may survey employees to discover their perceived needs and interests. Analysis of these data would indicate priority needs for health promotion programs.

College/University Setting. In the college or university setting, health education specialists are often involved in assessing student performance to meet state and national certification/licensure standards, as well as to meet program accreditation requirements. To revise curricula and meet accreditation standards, health education specialists track students' progress in meeting the standards, assess the learning environment, and analyze any links between the two.

College/University Health Services Setting. Health education specialists who practice in campus health services work closely with clinical practitioners in health, counseling, and fitness/wellness centers. Health education specialists assess the health needs of students, staff members, and faculty members through the use of focus groups, surveys, and interviews. In the assessment process, health education specialists develop avenues for obtaining information on knowledge, skills, perceptions, attitudes, beliefs, behaviors, learning preferences, and perceived needs in addition to health problems and practices. Once data are collected, health education specialists analyze them for factors that may impact the effectiveness of health education/promotion programs and interventions. The assessments form the basis of the priorities and recommendations for programs and interventions within the campus health services setting.

Section III: The HESPA 2015 Model

Table 3.2

Health Education Specialist Practice Analysis 2015 Model: Area of Responsibility I: Assess Needs, Resources, and Capacity for Health Education/Promotion

Area I: Assess Needs, Resources, and Capacity for Health Education/Promotion			
Competencies	Entry-level Sub-competencies	Advanced 1-level Sub-competencies	Advanced 2-level Sub-competencies
1.1 Plan assessment process for health education/promotion	1.1.1 Define the priority population to be assessed 1.1.2 Identify existing and necessary resources to conduct assessments 1.1.3 Engage priority populations, partners, and stakeholders to participate in the assessment process 1.1.5 Apply ethical principles to the assessment process	1.1.4 Apply theories and/or models to assessment process	
1.2 Access existing information and data related to health	1.2.1 Identify sources of secondary data related to health 1.2.3 Review related literature 1.2.4 Identify gaps in the secondary data 1.2.5 Extract data from existing databases 1.2.6 Determine the validity of existing data	1.2.2 Establish collaborative relationships and agreements that facilitate access to data	
1.3 Collect primary data to determine needs	1.3.1 Identify data collection instruments 1.3.2 Select data collection methods for use in assessment		

Section III: The HESPA 2015 Model

Area I: Assess Needs, Resources, and Capacity for Health Education/Promotion			
Competencies	Entry-level Sub-competencies	Advanced 1-level Sub-competencies	Advanced 2-level Sub-competencies
	1.3.3 Develop data collection procedures 1.3.4 Train personnel assisting with data collection 1.3.5 Implement quantitative and/or qualitative data collection		
1.4 Analyze relationships among behavioral, environmental, and other factors that influence health			
	1.4.1 Identify and analyze factors that influence health behaviors 1.4.2 Identify and analyze factors that impact health 1.4.3 Identify the impact of emerging social, economic, and other trends on health		
1.5 Examine factors that influence the process by which people learn			
	1.5.1 Identify and analyze factors that foster or hinder the learning process 1.5.2 Identify and analyze factors that foster or hinder knowledge acquisition 1.5.3 Identify and analyze factors that influence attitudes and beliefs 1.5.4 Identify and analyze factors that foster or hinder acquisition of skills		
1.6 Examine factors that enhance or impede the process of health education/promotion			
	1.6.1 Determine the extent of available health education/promotion programs and interventions		

Section III: The HESPA 2015 Model

Area I: Assess Needs, Resources, and Capacity for Health Education/Promotion			
Competencies	**Entry-level Sub-competencies**	**Advanced 1-level Sub-competencies**	**Advanced 2-level Sub-competencies**
	1.6.2 Identify policies related to health education/promotion 1.6.3 Assess the effectiveness of existing health education/promotion programs and interventions 1.6.4 Assess social, environmental, political, and other factors that may impact health education/promotion 1.6.5 Analyze the capacity for providing necessary health education/promotion		
1.7 Determine needs for health education/promotion based on assessment findings			
	1.7.2 Identify current needs, resources, and capacity 1.7.3 Prioritize health education/promotion needs 1.7.4 Develop recommendations for health education/promotion based on assessment findings 1.7.5 Report assessment findings	1.7.1 Synthesize assessment findings	

Section III: The HESPA 2015 Model

Area of Responsibility II: Plan Health Education/Promotion

The Role. Program planning begins once the assessment of existing needs, resources, and capacity has been completed. The planning process involves individuals from the priority population, program partners, and other stakeholders. After the planning group is formed, the members of the group work to develop program missions, goals, and objectives, as well as create or adapt intervention strategies, locate the resources needed to implement and evaluate the program, develop a plan for delivery, and address the factors that influence the implementation of the intervention. This time is also when health education specialists begin the planning process for program evaluation (see Table 3.3).

Settings. The following text is presented to describe how planning is used in different practice settings.

Community Setting. In a community setting where a needs assessment has been used to identify a significant health problem, the role of health education specialists is to convene representatives of relevant groups for the purpose of planning a health education/promotion program to address these needs. In identifying committee members, health education specialists may seek input and promote involvement from those who will affect, and be affected by, the program. Another key responsibility of health education specialists is to lead efforts to formulate goals and objectives and to develop evidence-based interventions that meet the needs of priority populations. Health education specialists identify and assess community resources and barriers affecting the implementation of the program to achieve a successful program or intervention in the community setting.

The selection of program activities and interventions depends on the characteristics of the priority population: its constraints, concerns, budget, timeframe, and the fit between program schedules and other obligations of the participants.

School (K-12) Setting. Administrators, public policy, or law usually make or mandate the decision to provide health education in schools. School health education specialists organize an advisory committee consisting of teachers, administrators, members of the community, representatives from voluntary agencies, parents, youth group leaders, clergy, and students to select and develop health education curricula and materials. These decisions are based on research results and best practices. The advisory committee may consider available resources and barriers to implementation, such as time and space, and objectives based on the needs of school-aged children and adolescents. Ultimately, the curricula follow a logical scope and sequence, as well as focus on maintaining or improving health behaviors.

Health Care Setting. Health education specialists in the health care setting work with nurses, physicians, nutritionists, physical therapists, patients, and other health care professionals to plan patient and community education programs. This team develops education programs for patients and their families to assist with decision-making, promote compliance with medical directions, and enhance understanding of medical procedures and conditions. The role of health education specialists in this setting is to assist the team in establishing goals and objectives, identifying staff member roles in providing education, selecting teaching methods and strategies, evaluating results, documenting the education effort, designing promotion activities, and training interdisciplinary staff to conduct the program.

Business/Industry Setting. In the workplace, health education specialists analyze data from numerous sources, including insurance and safety records, workers' compensation claims, and self-reported employee questionnaires. These data provide the basis for a presentation to management outlining the benefits and costs of a health education program. After gaining management's support, health education specialists convene an employee committee with representatives from all levels of the organization to develop a strategic plan outlining program priorities, goals and objectives, schedules, publicity strategies, incentives, and fees, as well as potential barriers and proposed solutions. Health education specialists lead the team in developing evidence-based interventions and strategies to meet the needs of employees.

College/University Setting. Health education specialists in a higher education setting analyze research results, current professional Competencies, accreditation standards, and certification requirements. Health education specialists use these results to design professional preparation programs that develop essential health education planning Competencies in candidates, regardless of their future practice setting.

College/University Health Services Setting. Using assessment results, health education specialists who practice in campus health services work closely with clinical practitioners in health, counseling, and fitness/wellness centers. This team works together to develop program goals and objectives, as well as to select and design strategies or interventions that address issues and improve health. Health education specialists develop partnerships with clinical practitioners, academicians, students, and others to integrate health education into other programs, including treatment regimens and campus wide activities. They also evaluate the efficacy of educational methods in achieving objectives.

Section III: The HESPA 2015 Model

Table 3.3

Health Education Specialist Practice Analysis 2015 Model: Area of Responsibility II: Plan Health Education/Promotion

Area II: Plan Health Education/Promotion			
Competencies	Entry-level Sub-competencies	Advanced 1-level Sub-competencies	Advanced 2-level Sub-competencies
2.1 Involve priority populations, partners, and other stakeholders in the planning process			
	2.1.1 Identify priority populations, partners, and other stakeholders 2.1.2 Use strategies to convene priority populations, partners, and other stakeholders 2.1.3 Facilitate collaborative efforts among priority populations, partners, and other stakeholders 2.1.4 Elicit input about the plan 2.1.5 Obtain commitments to participate in health education/promotion		
2.2 Develop goals and objectives			
	2.2.1 Identify desired outcomes using the needs assessment results 2.2.2 Develop vision statement 2.2.3 Develop mission statement 2.2.4 Develop goal statements 2.2.5 Develop specific, measurable, attainable, realistic, and time sensitive objectives		
2.3 Select or design strategies/interventions			
	2.3.4 Apply principles of cultural competence in selecting and/or designing strategies/interventions	2.3.1 Select planning model(s) for health education/promotion	

Section III: The HESPA 2015 Model

Area II: Plan Health Education/Promotion			
Competencies	**Entry-level Sub-competencies**	**Advanced 1-level Sub-competencies**	**Advanced 2-level Sub-competencies**
	2.3.5 Address diversity within priority populations in selecting and/or designing strategies/interventions 2.3.6 Identify delivery methods and settings to facilitate learning 2.3.7 Tailor strategies/interventions for priority populations 2.3.8 Adapt existing strategies/interventions as needed 2.3.11 Apply ethical principles in selecting strategies and designing interventions 2.3.12 Comply with legal standards in selecting strategies and designing interventions	2.3.2 Assess efficacy of various strategies/interventions to ensure consistency with objectives 2.3.3 Apply principles of evidence-based practice in selecting and/or designing strategies/interventions 2.3.9 Conduct pilot test of strategies/interventions 2.3.10 Refine strategies/interventions based on pilot feedback	
2.4 Develop a plan for the delivery of health education/promotion			
	2.4.1 Use theories and/or models to guide the delivery plan 2.4.2 Identify the resources involved in the delivery of health education/promotion 2.4.3 Organize health education/promotion into a logical sequence 2.4.4 Develop a timeline for the delivery of health education/promotion 2.4.5 Develop marketing plan to deliver health program 2.4.6 Select methods and/or channels for reaching priority populations		

Section III: The HESPA 2015 Model

Area II: Plan Health Education/Promotion			
Competencies	Entry-level Sub-competencies	Advanced 1-level Sub-competencies	Advanced 2-level Sub-competencies
	2.4.7 Analyze the opportunity for integrating health education/promotion into other programs 2.4.9 Assess the sustainability of the delivery plan 2.4.10 Design and conduct pilot study of health education/promotion plan	2.4.8 Develop a process for integrating health education/promotion into other programs when needed	
2.5 Address factors that influence implementation of health education/promotion			
	2.5.1 Identify and analyze factors that foster or hinder implementation 2.5.2 Develop plans and processes to overcome potential barriers to implementation		

Section III: The HESPA 2015 Model

Area of Responsibility III: Implement Health Education/Promotion

The Role. Health education specialists, regardless of the setting in which they work, implement planned programs to assist those in priority populations with maintaining or improving their health. To do so, health education specialists must coordinate the logistics to implement the plan, train volunteers and staff members involved in the implementation, deliver the program, monitor the progress of the program, and evaluate the sustainability of the program. Each of these steps must be completed while ensuring compliance with legal standards and while adhering to the ethical principles of the profession (see Table 3.4).

Settings. The following text is presented to describe how implementation is used in different practice settings.

Community Setting. Once a health education program has been created for a priority population, health education specialists must work to identify and obtain the resources to implement the program. Personnel are a primary resource in implementing any such program. Health education specialists will need to train staff members and volunteers or obtain assistance from a community coalition to implement the program. After launching the program, health education specialists continue to monitor progress and consider various strategies for sustaining the program over time.

School (K-12) Setting. In a school setting, health education specialists work to increase students' knowledge and to promote positive attitudes and behaviors regarding health. The school administration typically provides a curriculum to school-based health education specialists. From the curriculum, health education specialists infer objectives appropriate to students' learning potential and abilities, as well as decide on appropriate teaching techniques. Health education specialists' awareness of the students' learning needs, health behaviors, and related factors inform lesson plans. Health education specialists assess and monitor student learning to facilitate revisions in curricula and instructional methods, and also work with administrative staff members, faculty members, parent groups, and community groups to encourage school policies that support healthy behaviors.

Health Care Setting. Health education specialists employed in health care often serve as liaisons between patients and providers to enhance patient education. In addition, they can serve as outreach coordinators and provide patient education programs in the health care facility. Thus, health education specialists in this setting might conduct a program to support patients' weight-loss efforts. They may offer classes, supported by presentations from the health care providers and make use of educational materials consistent with the patients' needs. Health education specialists arrange opportunities to apply information learned through cooking classes or a grocery store tour to improve ability to read food labels. They may monitor participant outcomes and providers' reactions and the process of delivering such activities to make changes to the program and objectives as warranted.

Business/Industry Setting. In the workplace, health education specialists work with employers to offer educational programs that respond to employees' health and lifestyle needs in a manner conducive to employee participation. Health education specialists must understand the needs and interests of employees, the workplace culture, and the ways of doing business that might affect healthy behaviors. Health education specialists may offer healthful food choices in the company cafeteria, exercise classes, stress reduction counseling, and smoking cessation therapy, all supplemented by educational materials.

College/University Setting. Once a professional preparation program is created, health education specialists working in a higher education setting use their knowledge and skills to implement academic programs and prepare future health education specialists. Specifically, they use a variety of teaching methods, including lectures, discussions, simulations, practical experiences, and focused assignments. These methods and curricula help their students develop the essential health education implementation Competencies regardless of their future practice setting.

College/University Health Services Setting. In this setting, health education specialists work with others on campus to implement programs that address established needs utilizing best practices, appropriate theories, and a variety of strategies. Health education specialists may coordinate special events, develop health initiatives, arrange for screenings by other agencies, or develop programs for priority populations within the campus community. Program settings vary, and can include academic classrooms, residence halls, and fraternity/sorority meetings. For example, with the support of appropriate campus personnel, health education specialists may work with residence hall officials to offer educational sessions on several topics, including safer sex, alcohol and other drugs, relationship violence, stress and time management, smoking cessation, nutrition, and physical activity. Program availability must match student needs and be supported by media and activities intended to appeal to the college student. Health education specialists monitor program implementation, participant interest, and attendance, as well as request feedback to improve and direct future programming.

Section III: The HESPA 2015 Model

Table 3.4

Health Education Specialist Practice Analysis 2015 Model: Area of Responsibility III: Implement Health Education/Promotion

Area III: Implement Health Education/Promotion			
Competencies	**Entry-level Sub-competencies**	**Advanced 1-level Sub-competencies**	**Advanced 2-level Sub-competencies**
3.1 Coordinate logistics necessary to implement plan			
	3.1.1 Create an environment conducive to learning 3.1.2 Develop materials to implement plan 3.1.3 Secure resources to implement plan 3.1.4 Arrange for needed services to implement plan 3.1.5 Apply ethical principles to the implementation process 3.1.6 Comply with legal standards that apply to implementation		
3.2 Train staff members and volunteers involved in implementation of health education/promotion			
	3.2.2 Recruit individuals needed for implementation	3.2.1 Develop training objectives 3.2.3 Identify training needs of individuals involved in implementation 3.2.4 Develop training using best practices 3.2.5 Implement training 3.2.6 Provide support and technical assistance to those implementing the plan 3.2.7 Evaluate training 3.2.8 Use evaluation findings to plan/modify future training	

Section III: The HESPA 2015 Model

	Area III: Implement Health Education/Promotion		
Competencies	**Entry-level Sub-competencies**	**Advanced 1-level Sub-competencies**	**Advanced 2-level Sub-competencies**
3.3 Implement health education/promotion plan			
	3.3.1 Collect baseline data 3.3.3 Assess readiness for implementation 3.3.4 Apply principles of diversity and cultural competence in implementing health education/promotion plan 3.3.5 Implement marketing plan 3.3.6 Deliver health education/promotion as designed 3.3.7 Use a variety of strategies to deliver plan	3.3.2 Apply theories and/or models of implementation	
3.4 Monitor implementation of health education/promotion			
	3.4.1 Monitor progress in accordance with timeline 3.4.2 Assess progress in achieving objectives 3.4.3 Ensure plan is implemented consistently 3.4.4 Modify plan when needed 3.4.5 Monitor use of resources 3.4.6 Evaluate sustainability of implementation 3.4.7 Ensure compliance with legal standards 3.4.8 Monitor adherence to ethical principles in the implementation of health education/promotion		

Section III: The HESPA 2015 Model

Area of Responsibility IV: Conduct Evaluation and Research Related to Health Education/Promotion

The Role. The knowledge and skill sets necessary to conduct evaluation and research related to health education/promotion have much in common. Both research and evaluation require health education specialists to be competent in developing plans to guide their work. This includes selecting, adapting, and/or creating data collection instruments, as well as collecting and managing data, analyzing collected data, interpreting results, and applying the findings. These Competencies allow health education specialists to conduct evaluations of policy, projects, and programs, as well as to plan and conduct both basic and applied research. Health education specialists with advanced-level training and several years of experience working in the field complete much of this work because of the complexity of many of these processes (see Table 3.5).

Settings. The following text is presented to describe how research and evaluation are used in different practice settings.

Community Setting. Health education specialists in a community setting must understand and interpret research findings for use in their work. Their work may include the use of epidemiological principles to explain disease outbreaks or define high-risk neighborhoods within communities that require special program emphasis. Health education specialists must master research principles and language to discuss any topic important to the community, including unintentional injuries, an outbreak of measles or food poisoning, or sexually transmitted diseases. They also must understand the importance of conducting and interpreting the results of sound evaluations. Evaluations provide necessary evidence to support programs when reviewed by local or state governments. Health education specialists working at the entry-level may be involved in data collection for both research and evaluations, as well as interpreting the results of each of these processes. Those health education specialists working at an advanced-level of practice are responsible for planning and implementing the research and evaluation processes.

School (K-12) Setting. Health education specialists practicing in the school setting may be called upon to assist in the documentation of student health knowledge, attitudes, and behaviors. Health education specialists provide data gained from a review of the literature and from qualitative and quantitative research to school boards and parents to help them understand students' needs and interests. Careful use of such research approaches helps dispel intolerant attitudes and behaviors maintained by a small but vocal population. Evaluation of curriculum goals, objectives, learning activities, and behavioral outcomes is critical to identifying, selecting, and implementing effective curricula. As accountability increases, both qualitative and quantitative research methods are increasingly being emphasized in school settings.

Health Care Setting. In a health care setting, health education specialists must be able to understand and interpret research findings for patients and their families and may be asked to participate as a member of a research team that investigates behavioral components of adherence to clinical regimens. As medical technologies and treatments advance through clinical trials, evaluative research becomes increasingly important in addressing chronic disease conditions and the reduction of health risk behaviors for primary prevention. In addition, health education specialists may be involved in quality improvement initiatives as a member of the health care team.

Section III: The HESPA 2015 Model

Business/Industry Setting. Adults spend the majority of their time in the workplace. Health education specialists in this setting need qualitative and quantitative research skills to demonstrate the efficacy of health promotion programs and the contributions of such programs to productivity and organizational goals. Health education specialists also may be asked to assist in monitoring the work environment for safety compliance and injury reduction. Additionally, using evaluative research, health education specialists may be able to help determine quality and cost-effectiveness of competing health plans to benefit employers and employees.

College/University Setting. A significant portion of the work of health education specialists in this setting deals with both evaluation and research. As faculty members, health education specialists evaluate student work and teach students to apply research and evaluation Competencies in their future professional settings. These same health education specialists may also be contracted to serve as evaluators for community projects. They are expected to engage in scholarly endeavors that include research, grant proposal writing, and dissemination of research findings via publications and presentations. These efforts each contribute to the scientific body of knowledge encompassing health behavior, disease prevention, and risk reduction strategies, as well as to the profession of health education.

College/University Health Services Setting. Health education specialists working in the campus health services setting face many of the same issues as those in the business/industry and health care settings. These health education specialists need skills in all facets of research. Evaluative research skills are necessary to determine the efficacy and cost-effectiveness of programs for students, staff members, and faculty members. Health education specialists are expected to communicate findings and solicit feedback from stakeholders. Findings and feedback are incorporated into program/intervention improvement.

Section III: The HESPA 2015 Model

Table 3.5

Health Education Specialist Practice Analysis 2015 Model: Area of Responsibility IV: Conduct Evaluation and Research Related to Health Education/Promotion

Area IV: Conduct Evaluation and Research Related to Health Education/Promotion			
Competencies	Entry-level Sub-competencies	Advanced 1-level Sub-competencies	Advanced 2-level Sub-competencies
4.1 Develop evaluation plan for health education/ promotion		4.1.1 Determine the purpose and goals of evaluation 4.1.2 Develop questions to be answered by the evaluation 4.1.3 Create a logic model to guide the evaluation process 4.1.4 Adapt/modify a logic model to guide the evaluation process 4.1.5 Assess needed and available resources to conduct evaluation 4.1.6 Determine the types of data (for example, qualitative, quantitative) to be collected 4.1.7 Select a model for evaluation 4.1.8 Develop data collection procedures for evaluation 4.1.10 Apply ethical principles to the evaluation process	4.1.9 Develop data analysis plan for evaluation

Area IV: Conduct Evaluation and Research Related to Health Education/Promotion

Competencies	Entry-level Sub-competencies	Advanced 1-level Sub-competencies	Advanced 2-level Sub-competencies
4.2 Develop a research plan for health education/promotion			4.2.1 Create statement of purpose 4.2.2 Assess feasibility of conducting research 4.2.3 Conduct search for related literature 4.2.4 Analyze and synthesize information found in the literature 4.2.5 Develop research questions and/or hypotheses 4.2.6 Assess the merits and limitations of qualitative and quantitative data collection 4.2.7 Select research design to address the research questions 4.2.8 Determine suitability of existing data collection instruments 4.2.9 Identify research participants 4.2.10 Develop sampling plan to select participants 4.2.11 Develop data collection procedures for research 4.2.12 Develop data analysis plan for research 4.2.13 Develop a plan for nonrespondent follow up 4.2.14 Apply ethical principles to the research process

Section III: The HESPA 2015 Model

Area IV: Conduct Evaluation and Research Related to Health Education/Promotion			
Competencies	**Entry-level Sub-competencies**	**Advanced 1-level Sub-competencies**	**Advanced 2-level Sub-competencies**
4.3 Select, adapt, and/or create instruments to collect data			
	4.3.4 Identify useable items from existing instruments 4.3.5 Adapt/modify existing items		4.3.1 Identify existing data collection instruments 4.3.2 Adapt/modify existing data collection instruments 4.3.3 Create new data collection instruments 4.3.6 Create new items to be used in data collection 4.3.7 Pilot test data collection instrument 4.3.8 Establish validity of data collection instruments 4.3.9 Ensure that data collection instruments generate reliable data 4.3.10 Ensure fairness of data collection instruments (for example, reduce bias, use language appropriate to priority population)
4.4 Collect and manage data			
	4.4.3 Monitor and manage data collection 4.4.4 Use available technology to collect, monitor and manage data 4.4.5 Comply with laws and regulations when collecting, storing, and protecting participant data		4.4.1 Train data collectors involved in evaluation and/or research 4.4.2 Collect data based on the evaluation or research plan
4.6 Interpret results			
		4.5.2 Analyze data using qualitative methods	4.5.1 Prepare data for analysis

Section III: The HESPA 2015 Model

Area IV: Conduct Evaluation and Research Related to Health Education/Promotion			
Competencies	Entry-level Sub-competencies	Advanced 1-level Sub-competencies	Advanced 2-level Sub-competencies
			4.5.3 Analyze data using descriptive statistical methods
			4.5.4 Analyze data using inferential statistical methods
			4.5.5 Use technology to analyze data
4.6 Interpret results			
			4.6.1 Synthesize the analyzed data
			4.6.2 Explain how the results address the questions and/or hypotheses
			4.6.3 Compare findings to results from other studies or evaluations
			4.6.4 Propose possible explanations of findings
			4.6.5 Identify limitations of findings
			4.6.6 Address delimitations as they relate to findings
			4.6.7 Draw conclusions based on findings
			4.6.8 Develop recommendations based on findings
4.7 Apply findings			
	4.7.1 Communicate findings to priority populations, partners, and stakeholders		4.7.5 Disseminate findings using a variety of methods
	4.7.2 Solicit feedback from priority populations, partners, and stakeholders		
	4.7.3 Evaluate feasibility of implementing recommendations		
	4.7.4 Incorporate findings into program improvement and refinement		

Section III: The HESPA 2015 Model

Area of Responsibility V: Administer and Manage Health Education/Promotion

The Role. Health education/promotion programs must not only be planned and implemented well but also administered and managed well once launched. While some administrative (i.e., gaining program support) and managerial (i.e., managing technological resources) functions may fall to the entry-level health education specialist, administration and management is generally a function of the more advanced-level practitioner. Health education specialists often become program managers or supervisors of other health education specialists and/or teams of allied health professionals. Good management incorporates effective leadership skills with managing financial, technological, and human resources. Successful managers maintain relationships with partners and other stakeholders, assign tasks, and conduct performance evaluations. Supervisors facilitate discussions with both internal and external stakeholders such as advanced-level management as well as funding agencies in regards to program resource needs. This role requires effective communication skills, organizational knowledge, and objectivity. Because of their broad training and their understanding of individuals and communities, health education specialists can be effective managers who consider potential partnerships in the larger context of their institution and environment (see Table 3.6).

Settings. The following text is presented to describe how administering programs is used in different practice settings.

Community Setting. Health education specialists in a community setting, especially those working at an advanced-level, may be responsible for managing and administering health education/promotion programs. Such work includes gaining acceptance for programs and managing the financial, technological, and human resources associated with programs. These tasks require health education specialists to create and monitor a program budget, hire and evaluate personnel, and work with both internal and external partners, as well as stakeholders, to ensure a program's success. In addition, health education specialists are responsible for managing the relationships with program partners and other stakeholders.

School (K-12) Setting. In addition to managing students in the classroom, health education specialists in the school setting must identify and secure financial resources to support program and policy changes that help improve students' learning and health. Health education specialists serve as curriculum coordinators or project directors, manage curricular and budgetary issues for the school health program, and work with school health advisory councils to obtain acceptance and support for content areas addressed in the curriculum. Health education specialists also frequently supervise pre-service interns (student teachers). As curriculum specialists or program heads, they serve as team leaders to promote health education in their school, throughout the school district, and at the state level.

Health Care Settings. Health education specialists may manage professional development programs in medical complexes, nursing homes, or transitional facilities. The ability to communicate and facilitate partnerships with a variety of medical professionals, aides, volunteers, patients, family, or community members is very important in this setting. Planning programs that contribute to institutional maintenance of accreditation and compliance with government regulations also may be the task of health education specialists.

Section III: The HESPA 2015 Model

These health education specialists may supervise institutional service learning activities that augment staff efforts.

Business/Industry Setting. In this setting, health education specialists may lead or be part of a team as either a coordinator for an employee assistance program or director of a health promotion effort. As employees, health education specialists also may supervise or provide support for employed staff members, contracted staff members, vendors, or volunteers in health promotion programs (e.g., smoking cessation, stress management, substance misuse, and weight loss).

College/University Setting. Health education specialists in the college/university setting may be involved in a variety of administrative responsibilities, including coordinating professional preparation programs and chairing academic departments. In this role, health education specialists must develop and manage program budgets, supervise part-time faculty members, and be responsible for the annual evaluations of those employed in the department. They also must align their professional preparation program goals with the goals and mission of college/university. In addition, health education specialists may coordinate and supervise student internships, analyze the program's curriculum for appropriate goals and objectives, and chair or facilitate committees. In this setting, health education specialists also must teach administration and management Competencies to students in their professional preparation program.

College/University Health Services Setting. Health education specialists in a campus health services setting may coordinate special events, develop health initiatives, arrange for health screenings by other agencies, or develop health education programs for priority populations within the community. These same health education specialists also may administer health education/promotion programs, as well as health, counseling, or fitness/wellness services centers. In this role, they must demonstrate leadership, plan strategically, and organize the center. Health education specialists also must hire, administer, train, manage, and evaluate personnel, as well as secure funds and manage financial, technological, and other resources. In addition, they advocate for support and acceptance of health education/promotion programs, conduct quality assurance, process improvement studies, facilitate organizational change, and manage stakeholder relationships.

Section III: The HESPA 2015 Model

Table 3.6

Health Education Specialists Practice Analysis 2015 Model: Area of Responsibility V: Administer and Manage Health Education/Promotion

Area V: Administer and Manage Health Education/Promotion			
Competencies	**Entry-level Sub-competencies**	**Advanced 1-level Sub-competencies**	**Advanced 2-level Sub-competencies**
5.1 Manage financial resources for health education/promotion programs			
		5.1.1 Develop financial plan 5.1.2 Evaluate financial needs and resources 5.1.3 Identify internal and/or external funding sources 5.1.4 Prepare budget requests 5.1.5 Develop program budgets 5.1.6 Manage program budgets 5.1.7 Conduct cost analysis for programs 5.1.8 Prepare budget reports 5.1.9 Monitor financial plan 5.1.10 Create requests for funding proposals 5.1.11 Write grant proposals 5.1.12 Conduct reviews of funding proposals 5.1.13 Apply ethical principles when managing financial resources	

Section III: The HESPA 2015 Model

Area V: Administer and Manage Health Education/Promotion			
Competencies	**Entry-level Sub-competencies**	**Advanced 1-level Sub-competencies**	**Advanced 2-level Sub-competencies**
5.2 Manage technology resources			
	5.2.1 Assess technology needs to support health education/promotion 5.2.2 Use technology to collect, store, and retrieve program management data 5.2.3 Apply ethical principles in managing technology resources 5.2.4 Evaluate emerging technologies for applicability to health education/promotion		
5.3 Manage relationships with partners and other stakeholders			
	5.3.1 Assess capacity of partners and other stakeholders to meet program goals 5.3.3 Create agreements (for example, memoranda of understanding) with partners and other stakeholders 5.3.4 Monitor relationships with partners and other stakeholders 5.3.6 Evaluate relationships with partners and other stakeholders	5.3.2 Facilitate discussions with partners and other stakeholders regarding program resource needs 5.3.5 Elicit feedback from partners and other stakeholders	
5.4 Gain acceptance and support for health education/promotion programs			
	5.4.1 Demonstrate how programs align with organizational structure, mission, and goals 5.4.2 Identify evidence to justify programs 5.4.3 Create a rationale to gain or maintain program support 5.4.4 Use various communication strategies to present rationale		

Section III: The HESPA 2015 Model

Area V: Administer and Manage Health Education/Promotion			
Competencies	**Entry-level Sub-competencies**	**Advanced 1-level Sub-competencies**	**Advanced 2-level Sub-competencies**
5.5 Demonstrate leadership	5.5.2 Analyze an organization's culture to determine the extent to which it supports health education/promotion 5.5.3 Develop strategies to reinforce or change organizational culture to support health education/promotion 5.5.8 Conduct program quality assurance/process improvement 5.5.9 Comply with existing laws and regulations 5.5.10 Adhere to ethical principles of the profession	5.5.1 Facilitate efforts to achieve organizational mission 5.5.4 Facilitate needed changes to organizational culture 5.5.5 Conduct strategic planning 5.5.6 Implement strategic plan 5.5.7 Monitor strategic plan	
5.6 Manage human resources for health education/promotion programs	5.6.5 Recruit staff members and volunteers for programs	5.6.1 Assess staffing needs 5.6.2 Develop job descriptions 5.6.3 Apply human resource policies consistent with laws and regulations 5.6.4 Evaluate qualifications of staff members and volunteers needed for programs 5.6.6 Determine staff member and volunteer professional development needs 5.6.7 Develop strategies to enhance staff member and volunteer professional development	

Section III: The HESPA 2015 Model

Area V: Administer and Manage Health Education/Promotion			
Competencies	**Entry-level Sub-competencies**	**Advanced 1-level Sub-competencies**	**Advanced 2-level Sub-competencies**
		5.6.8 Implement strategies to enhance the professional development of staff members and volunteers	
		5.6.9 Develop and implement strategies to retain staff members and volunteers	
		5.6.10 Employ conflict resolution techniques	
		5.6.11 Facilitate team development	
		5.6.12 Evaluate performance of staff members and volunteers	
		5.6.13 Monitor performance and/or compliance of funding recipients	
		5.6.14 Apply ethical principles when managing human resources	

Section III: The HESPA 2015 Model

Area of Responsibility VI: Serve as a Health Education/Promotion Resource Person

The Role. The setting in which health education specialists function largely determines the nature of the resources provided for a program. When requested, health education specialists need to serve as a resource for valid health information and materials. They must be aware of a variety of community resources at the local, state, and national levels as well as familiar with online databases and able to evaluate the accuracy, relevance, and timeliness of resource materials. In addition, health education specialists must be able to adapt health related information for, and to, those in the priority population. Finally, health education specialists practicing at the advanced-level need to train others to use health education/promotion skills, assess and prioritize requests for advice and consultation, and establish advisory and consultative relationships, as well as provide and evaluate the effects of expert assistance and guidance (see Table 3.7).

Settings. The following text is presented to describe how acting as a resource is used in different practice settings.

Community Setting. Health education specialists serving as resource persons in a community setting may be asked to assist community-based organizations, local voluntary health organizations, churches, civic organizations, neighborhood associations, and other nonprofits. In this capacity, health education specialists might be asked to provide current health information (i.e., suggestions on relevant literature findings, audiovisual materials, educational pamphlets, and posters for distribution) and serve on various community-wide coalitions to help identify and implement strategies to improve health. They also may be called on to train others to better plan, implement, and evaluate health education/promotion programs. Those health education specialists practicing at an advanced-level may serve as advisors or consultants for new community organizations just beginning to offer health education/promotion programs.

School (K-12) Setting. Health education specialists in the school setting may participate in the work of a curriculum committee formed to identify and select educational materials in compliance with state legislative mandates and school district policies. Health education specialists provide expert assistance to committee members in examining state laws and codes, establishing criteria for the evaluation of instructional materials, and recommending placement of the topic in the overall curriculum scope and sequence plan. After selecting the material, health education specialists arrange preview sessions for interested parents and community members.

Health Care Setting. Health care settings may include hospitals, medical centers, clinics, and satellite clinics. Health education specialists in these health care settings serve as consultants to a community group by developing chronic disease prevention and control education programs. Health education specialists provide information on successful or evidence-based programs, help identify culturally and linguistically appropriate materials, conduct focus groups to assist in planning interventions, identify expert speakers, and help identify media and other communication channels for disseminating information about the program to the community. These health education specialists also may facilitate use of community services by providing links to health care services and the community.

Section III: The HESPA 2015 Model

Business/Industry Setting. Physical fitness, stress management, and nutrition programs are frequently featured in worksite health education/promotion programming. As resource persons, health education specialists are responsible for disseminating information to employers and employees about these programs in a timely manner. Health education specialists identify and organize resources needed for the implementation and continuation of health education/promotion programs and policy changes at the worksite to promote health. They also identify data to present to key personnel and monitor the plans of those responsible for conducting the program in order to ensure that activities match the stated goals, objectives, and budget. In addition, health education specialists identify and/or develop relevant health promotion materials about specific topics to display and distribute to employees at the worksite.

College/University Setting. Health education specialists often serve as consultants to community agencies and local school districts. In that role, they often provide and share health education/promotion resources and information. Health education specialists must be able to teach students how and where to obtain valid and reliable health information so that students may serve as resource persons in their future professional endeavors.

College/University Health Services Setting. Health education specialists in the campus health services setting serve as health education/promotion resources for the campus community. This role includes assessing needs for health information, evaluating resources, and adapting materials for the campus community. Some health education specialists may train others to use health education/promotion skills, as well as consult and advise on campus health issues.

Section III: The HESPA 2015 Model

Table 3.7

Health Education Specialist Practice Analysis 2015 Model: Area of Responsibility VI: Serve as a Health Education/Promotion Resource Person

Area VI: Serve as a Health Education/Promotion Resource Person			
Competencies	**Entry-level Sub-competencies**	**Advanced 1-level Sub-competencies**	**Advanced 2-level Sub-competencies**
6.1 Obtain and disseminate health related information	6.1.1 Assess needs for health related information 6.1.2 Identify valid information resources 6.1.3 Evaluate resource materials for accuracy, relevance, and timeliness 6.1.4 Adapt information for consumer 6.1.5 Convey health related information to consumer		
6.2 Train others to use health education/ promotion skills		6.2.1 Assess training needs of potential participants 6.2.2 Develop a plan for conducting training 6.2.3 Identify resources needed to conduct training 6.2.4 Implement planned training 6.2.5 Conduct formative and summative evaluations of training 6.2.6 Use evaluative feedback to create future trainings	

Section III: The HESPA 2015 Model

Area VI: Serve as a Health Education/Promotion Resource Person			
Competencies	**Entry-level Sub-competencies**	**Advanced 1-level Sub-competencies**	**Advanced 2-level Sub-competencies**
6.3 Provide advice and consultation on health education/promotion issues			
		6.3.1 Assess and prioritize requests for advice/consultation 6.3.2 Establish advisory/consultative relationships 6.3.3 Provide expert assistance and guidance 6.3.4 Evaluate the effectiveness of the expert assistance provided 6.3.5 Apply ethical principles in consultative relationships	

Section III: The HESPA 2015 Model

Area of Responsibility VII: Communicate, Promote, and Advocate for Health, Health Education/Promotion, and the Profession

The Role. Health education specialists are charged with the responsibility of providing information to diverse audiences. Whether through individual, small group, or mass communication strategies and techniques, health education specialists use their professional background to create, tailor, pilot test, deliver, and evaluate the impact of their communication. Their ability to communicate effectively provides health education specialists with the foundation to advocate for health and health education/promotion. As advocates, they create, implement, and evaluate plans that influence both policy and systems. Health education specialists' advocacy efforts also promote the profession of health education/promotion by explaining the history of the profession, the major responsibilities of health education specialists, and the role of professional organizations and credentialing in advancing the profession (Table 3.8).

Settings. The following text is used to describe how communication and advocacy are used in different health education practice settings.

Community Setting. In a community setting, health education specialists develop communication messages to be delivered through a variety of channels and program materials in the language of the priority population and at appropriate reading levels. Health education specialists also act as advocates for community health needs. Such advocates may lobby the local government to use funds in ways that help promote the community's health or create policy that promotes community health. Additionally, health education specialists promote the health education/promotion profession through service and mentorship.

School (K-12) Setting. When employed in a school setting, health education specialists may promote the Whole School, Whole Community, Whole Child (WSCC) model by presenting curriculum information and student health information needs and/or concerns to groups of parents. In the event of parental concerns, health education specialists must consider the multiple value systems represented by the group and employ appropriate strategies to communicate the material and respond to parents' questions. Depending on the topic, health education specialists may use illustrations from classroom instruction, student presentations, videos, or Web technology to enhance the presentation. Health education specialists also can advocate for students' and/or faculty members' health in a school setting by creating school health councils or teaching advocacy skills in the curriculum.

Health Care Setting. In this setting, health education specialists are often responsible for creating and updating all patient education materials. These materials include brochures, posters, flyers, public service announcements, and the health care facility's Web site. Health education specialists often serve as the voice for patient education and must advocate for its inclusion in the health care setting. Health education specialists also work with others in the health care system to ensure that the patient education materials are consistent throughout the system. Like health education specialists in other settings, health education specialists in this setting promote the health education/promotion profession through service and participation in professional health education organizations.

Business/Industry Setting. Health education specialists in the workplace might become aware of previously unrecognized health needs among employees. Health education specialists must

Section III: The HESPA 2015 Model

communicate those needs (e.g., insufficient opportunity for physical activity) to management. Using their background in behavioral and biological sciences, health education specialists interpret the problem for management and articulate the possible ways of addressing the problem, such as offering a program or screening or changing organizational policy. Health education specialists must acknowledge concerns specific to management to communicate ways in which a specific health education program or policy might benefit management and employees.

College/University Setting. Health education specialists in a college/university setting may face the challenge of ensuring health education's place in the college/university curricula. Communication supporting the program might be handled through reports to curricula committees, presentations to administrators, electronic communications, or small group discussions with members and students. University health education specialists may develop advocacy plans for improving the health of current and future students. They also teach their students how to communicate, promote, and advocate for health and health education. Beyond the university, health education specialists need to advocate for various community, state, and national health issues, as well as for the health education profession as a whole. Advocating may involve population-based strategies and the use of various media and social media outlets.

College/University Health Services Setting. In this setting, heath education specialists utilize a variety of communication techniques and technology platforms to develop, evaluate, and deliver messages to the campus community. These messages may be advocating for resources, policy, and system changes to improve health or promote the profession. Health education specialists must explain their role on campus relative to other areas, the benefits of participating in professional organizations, and how to become credentialed. Communication, promotion, and advocacy intersect in the college/university setting. For example, health education specialists may be responsible for implementing a social norm campaign to improve students' decisions concerning the use of alcohol and other drugs. They must communicate the need for the campaign to stakeholders. These needs may include the educational purpose, relevant social norms data, and an interpretation of the program's value relative to the established needs and concerns of the community. This communication may be distributed via electronic or print channels (e.g., posters placed around campus, social media postings), as well as face-to-face (i.e., presentations to stakeholder groups). Health education specialists also work with select student organizations to encourage policy development regarding alcohol consumption on campus and alternatives to alcohol. They also may advocate for local laws or ordinances that strengthen alcohol or drug related offenses for businesses.

Section III: The HESPA 2015 Model

Table 3.8

Health Education Specialist Analysis 2015 Model: Area of Responsibility VII: Communicate, Promote, and Advocate for Health, Health Education/Promotion, and the Profession

Area VII: Communicate, Promote, and Advocate for Health, Health Education/Promotion, and the Profession			
Competencies	**Entry-level Sub-competencies**	**Advanced 1-level Sub-competencies**	**Advanced 2-level Sub-competencies**
7.1 Identify, develop, and deliver messages using a variety of communication strategies, methods, and techniques			
	7.1.1 Create messages using communication theories and/or models 7.1.2 Identify level of literacy of intended audience 7.1.3 Tailor messages for intended audience 7.1.6 Assess and select methods and technologies used to deliver messages 7.1.7 Deliver messages using media and communication strategies 7.1.8 Evaluate the impact of the delivered messages	7.1.4 Pilot test messages and delivery methods 7.1.5 Revise messages based on pilot feedback	
7.2 Engage in advocacy for health and health education/promotion			
	7.2.1 Identify current and emerging issues requiring advocacy 7.2.2 Engage stakeholders in advocacy initiatives 7.2.3 Access resources (for example, financial, personnel, information, data) related to identified advocacy needs 7.2.4 Develop advocacy plans in compliance with local, state, and/or federal policies and procedures		

Section III: The HESPA 2015 Model

Area VII: Communicate, Promote, and Advocate for Health, Health Education/Promotion, and the Profession

Competencies	Entry-level Sub-competencies	Advanced 1-level Sub-competencies	Advanced 2-level Sub-competencies
	7.2.5 Use strategies that advance advocacy goals 7.2.6 Implement advocacy plans 7.2.7 Evaluate advocacy efforts 7.2.8 Comply with organizational policies related to participating in advocacy 7.2.9 Lead advocacy initiatives related to health		
7.3 Influence policy and/or systems change to promote health and health education/promotion			
	7.3.1 Assess the impact of existing and proposed policies on health 7.3.2 Assess the impact of existing and proposed policies on health education 7.3.3 Assess the impact of existing systems on health 7.3.4 Project the impact of proposed systems changes on health education 7.3.5 Use evidence-based findings in policy analysis 7.3.9 Use media advocacy techniques to influence decision makers 7.3.10 Engage in legislative advocacy	7.3.6 Develop policies to promote health using evidence-based findings 7.3.7 Identify factors that influence decision makers 7.3.8 Use policy advocacy techniques to influence decision makers	
7.4 Promote the health education profession			
	7.4.1 Explain the major responsibilities of the health education specialist		7.4.9 Serve as a mentor to others in the profession

Section III: The HESPA 2015 Model

Area VII: Communicate, Promote, and Advocate for Health, Health Education/Promotion, and the Profession			
Competencies	**Entry-level Sub-competencies**	**Advanced 1-level Sub-competencies**	**Advanced 2-level Sub-competencies**
	7.4.2 Explain the role of professional organizations in advancing the profession 7.4.3 Explain the benefits of participating in professional organizations 7.4.4 Advocate for professional development of health education specialists 7.4.5 Advocate for the profession 7.4.6 Explain the history of the profession and its current and future implications for professional practice 7.4.7 Explain the role of credentialing (for example, individual, program) in the promotion of the profession 7.4.8 Develop and implement a professional development plan		7.4.10 Develop materials that contribute to the professional literature 7.4.11 Engage in service to advance the profession

This page was
intentionally left blank

Section IV: Using the HESPA 2015 Model

The HESPA 2015 is the fourth analysis of its kind to assure that qualified health education specialists have the knowledge and skills to educate the public. The first role delineation study was conducted from 1978 to 1981 and formed the basis for professional preparation, professional development, and the CHES examination (Cleary, 1995). Next, from the CUP Model (NCHEC, SOPHE, & AAHE, 2006), common standards of practice were established in a hierarchical framework for health education specialists. Soon after the HEJA 2010 (NCHEC, SOPHE, & AAHE, 2010) followed. A variety of stakeholders used these models to more clearly define, develop, and apply the Competencies and Sub-competencies of the profession. Like the HEJA 2010 Model, the HESPA 2015 Model serves the profession in a number of ways. However, the HESPA 2015 Model includes the newly-validated Seven Areas of Responsibility and 36 Competencies, as well as 141 entry-level, 76 advanced 1-level, and 41 advanced 2-level Sub-competencies. The HESPA Model also includes 131 verified specific knowledge items used by health education specialists. The following text is presented to describe the potential applications and benefits of the HESPA 2015 Model for selected stakeholder groups, including a set of formal recommendations to the profession endorsed by the boards of SOPHE, NCHEC, and CNHEO.

Health Education Students

Often students find choosing a career path in health education to be a confusing process. This confusion may be particularly true for individuals entering a university system for the first time with limited experience of the work settings associated with the wide variety of health education career options. Like its predecessors, the HESPA 2015 Model offers useful information to students interested in a career in health education, including a basic understanding of the Competencies and Sub-competencies commonly used by health education specialists. The HESPA 2015 Model also serves as a guide for students exploring the various work settings in which this understanding might be applied. Students considering a graduate degree in health education are better prepared to make the decision and choose a program if they are familiar with the entry- and advanced-level distinctions in the Model. The Model also allows students to compare the stated competencies in other professions and understand professional distinctions in general.

Students enrolled in health education degree programs may use the Model as a guide for self-directed learning and assessment. Moreover, the Model may help students set personal achievement goals specific to each Area of Responsibility and, subsequently, to assess progress toward mastery of each Area. Students may use the Competencies and Sub-competencies as a guide for selecting and evaluating degree programs and specific courses, as well as for actively seeking opportunities to serve as volunteers, interns, and/or employees to gain experience in a specific Area of Responsibility. The Model may be used as a framework in preparing for the national examination to become a CHES or MCHES. The framework also helps to create professional portfolios and résumés that reflect experiences and demonstrated abilities relevant to the profession.

College and University Faculty Members

Faculty members of health education professional preparation programs may use the HESPA 2015 Model for curriculum development, student mentorship, and program accreditation efforts. A Competency-based approach to curriculum development can enhance the marketability of program graduates and is an established standard for achieving formal approval/accreditation for health education programs. Faculty members and their students

Section IV: Using the HESPA 2015 Model

may benefit when expectations for student performance, faculty members' teaching, and mentorship are clearly defined within the Model framework. The Model is useful in developing program goals and objectives, course descriptions, syllabi and evaluation instruments, student handbooks, and specific guides for practica/internships, as well as portfolios and assessment tools for program approval and accreditation. The Model also may help faculty members to compare the stated competencies of other professional degrees offered by a university and develop program descriptions and marketing materials. Furthermore, the Model can serve as a guide for faculty members to communicate program needs to university administrators and to leverage resources and opportunities for program development. Faculty members are encouraged to seek and maintain approval/accreditation relevant to their degree programs and to conduct periodic reviews to assess and maintain relevance and currency in their programs (see Appendix D for matrices for analyzing curricula).

Health Education Practitioners
Practicing health education specialists may use the HESPA 2015 Model as a guide for professional development. Continuing education is not only a requirement for CHES and MCHES certifications but also essential for a practicing health education specialist to remain current, effective, and marketable in the field. The HESPA 2015 Model is useful in helping practitioners monitor changes in Competencies and Sub-competencies as they emerge, self-assess areas of needed renewal and new skill development, and select professional development opportunities directed toward current practices in the profession. Practitioners who are interested in changing work settings and/or being promoted to more advanced-levels of practice will be better equipped to do so if they are aware of and skilled in the generic entry-level and relevant advanced-level Competencies represented in the Model.

Professional Development Providers
Leaders of organizations and agencies that provide continuing education and professional development opportunities will benefit from using the HESPA 2015 Model as a guide. For example, health education specialists often look to these organizations and agencies as a source for staying current in an evolving professional field. As the number of CHES and MCHES continue to grow, the demand for Competency-based professional development opportunities will increase. Opportunities to renew and develop new skills represented in the HESPA 2015 Model will be critical to the future of a growing and evolving health education profession.

Other Health Professionals
The previously established CUP and HEJA 2010 Models have contributed to a growing understanding and appreciation for health education specialists among members of other health professions. Likewise, the HESPA 2015 Model can be used to further promote the growing appreciation for health education specialists and their valuable roles in health-related partnerships. It is a very concrete way to show others what health education specialists can contribute to helping others improve and maintain their health.

Health Education Employers
Most Competencies used by health education specialists are adaptable to a variety of work-related projects. Some Competencies enable a health education specialist to connect other health education specialists and communities together, as well as to achieve objectives in health promoting partnerships.

Section IV: Using HESPA 2015 Model

The HESPA 2015 Model contains an updated, empirically verified description of current practice at three levels and supports an appreciation for and employment of health education specialists. Employers are encouraged to use the HESPA 2015 Model when developing position announcements and job descriptions, supporting and requiring professional development for their employed health education specialists, and evaluating employee performance. CHES and MCHES credentials reflect mastery of current entry- and advanced-level Areas of Responsibility, Competencies, and Sub-competencies. In addition, employers are encouraged to employ individuals with these certifications.

Leaders of Professional Credentialing and Program Accreditation

The HESPA 2015 Model serves as the standard for individual credentialing and program approval or accreditation. The HESPA 2015 Model contains some different Sub-competencies and Competencies than the CUP or HEJA 2010 Models and, therefore, requires the development of specific items for the current CHES and MCHES examinations, as well as adjustments to criteria for program approval and accreditation. These changes enhance the profession's ability to assess and promote individual Competencies and program quality based on a more precise and expanded definition of Competencies and Sub-competencies. Inclusion of the entry-level Competencies at all levels of credentialing and accreditation and the addition of the advanced-level Competencies in criteria used for advanced-level credentialing and professional preparation will be important.

Policy Makers and Funding Agencies

Policy makers may use the HESPA 2015 Model in governmental and nongovernmental settings to establish organizational policies related to health education efforts. These policies often impact the development of health programs and interventions, as well as the criteria for funding projects and research. The Competencies and Sub-competencies further clarify the distinctive role of health education specialists at entry- and advanced-levels of practice. The United States Department of Labor and the states implementing the Standard Occupational Classification system should use the HESPA 2015 Model to collect data and monitor the job outlook for health education specialists.

Recommendations to the Profession

The HESPA 2015 outcomes have significant implications for professional preparation, certification, continuing education, and practice in the health education profession. In 2014, the boards of SOPHE and NCHEC issued seven recommendations for using the HESPA 2015 Model. In the same year when the recommendations were made, CNHEO also endorsed them. The recommendations build on earlier studies and reports for the field and reaffirm the following key principles: (a) health education is a single profession with common roles and responsibilities; (b) professional preparation in health education provides a health education specialist with knowledge and skills that form a foundation of generic Competencies; (c) accreditation is the primary quality assurance mechanism in higher education; and (d) the health education profession is responsible for assuring quality in professional preparation and practice.

To continue to advance the profession, the following recommendations (NCHEC & SOPHE, 2014) should provide a basis and direction for all future efforts:

Section IV: Using the HESPA 2015 Model

1. Baccalaureate degree programs with a health education emphasis should prepare graduates to perform all entry-level Competencies and Sub-competencies within the Areas of Responsibility. Additionally, curriculum should incorporate the verified knowledge items.

2. NCHEC should use all entry-level Competencies and Sub-competencies within the Areas of Responsibility as the basis for the Certified Health Education Specialist (CHES) examination. Additionally, examination questions should incorporate the verified knowledge items.

3. Master and doctoral programs with a health education emphasis should prepare graduates to perform all entry- and advanced-level Competencies and Sub-competencies within the Areas of Responsibility. Curricula should incorporate the verified knowledge items. Additionally, doctoral programs should prepare graduates to demonstrate a high level of competency and complexity in all advanced 2-level Sub-competencies.

4. NCHEC should use all entry- and advanced-level Competencies and Sub-competencies within the Areas of Responsibility as the basis for the advanced-level Master Certified Health Education Specialist (MCHES) examination. Additionally, examination questions should incorporate the verified knowledge items.

5. All entry- and advanced-level Competencies and Sub-competencies within the Areas of Responsibility and the verified knowledge items should serve as the basis for professional development and continuing education for the health education profession.

6. Accrediting agencies and approval bodies should be encouraged to recognize the Areas of Responsibility, Competencies, and Sub-competencies as the basis for quality assurance for health education professional preparation programs.

7. The HESPA hierarchical Model should be used as the basis for communicating about the Responsibilities and Competencies of the health education profession to public and private employers, national/state/local policymakers, health insurers, health professionals, and other stakeholders.

Profession-wide support of these seven recommendations can significantly impact the future of the health education profession. For example, NCHEC leaders are using the HESPA 2015 Model and verified knowledge items to update the CHES and MCHES examinations. The HESPA 2015 Model is also useful in coordinating the approach to accreditation for professional preparation programs. Professional development and continuing education opportunities may be planned for the three different levels of practice. As with previous practices analyses, the HESPA 2015 Model serves as a guide for future Competency updates. The regular, periodic revalidation of the health education Areas of Responsibility, Competencies, and Sub-competencies is a necessary process to ensure that certification, preparation, and professional development are based on the needs of current practice. Ideally this revalidation process will be completed every five years.

Section V: Changes in the Area of Responsibility: Competencies and Sub-competencies of Health Education Specialists from 1985 to 2015

This 2015 publication marks the 30th year since the first publication of the Seven Areas of Responsibility, which signified the first established role of entry-level health education specialists and the related scope of their practice. The HESPA 2015 Model presents the third series of changes made to that original framework to adapt to emerging changes in current practice, though the original Seven Areas of Responsibility remain largely intact. Table 5.1 illustrates how the profession began with Seven Areas of Responsibility in 1985, added three graduate-level areas (i.e., Areas VIII-X) in 1999, and then combined the original Seven Areas of Responsibility from 1985 and three graduate-level Areas from 1999 into an updated Seven Areas of Responsibility in 2006, and further refined the Seven Areas Responsibility once again in 2010. The revalidated Seven Areas of Responsibility in the HESPA 2015 Model are also provided in Table 5.1. As stated by the CUP Model authors, this constant in health education practice "is a testament to the solid foundations on which the profession stands" (NCHEC, SOPHE, & AAHE, 2006, p. 48).

The three-tiered hierarchical framework of entry- and advanced-level practice that emerged in the CUP Model has now been revalidated twice through the HEJA 2010 and HESPA 2015 Models, along with a large number of Competencies and Sub-competencies. However, as was true regarding earlier study outcomes, outcomes of the HESPA 2015 Model reveal the need for wording changes, the reassignment of some Competencies and Sub-competencies, and the addition of new Competencies and Sub-competencies to more accurately reflect the evolving practice of entry- and advanced-level health education specialists. The new numbering system to identify Responsibilities, Competencies, and Sub-competencies (see Section III) incorporates additional changes noted in the Model and descriptions below. These descriptions include a brief overview of changes made in the HESPA 2015 Model compared to the HEJA 2010 Model. A more detailed analysis of these changes appears in the grid provided in Appendix B titled, "Comparison of the Areas of Responsibility, Competencies, and Sub-competencies of the HEJA 2010 Model and the HESPA 2015 Model."

Seven Areas of Responsibility
The outcomes of the HESPA 2015 Model validate the continued use of the Seven Areas of Responsibility as established in both the HEJA 2010 and CUP Models. However, some revisions of the wording of the Areas of Responsibility were necessary. The two most notable changes are: (a) adding the word *promotion* to each of the Seven Areas of Responsibility to replace the term *health education* with *health education/promotion*, and (b) expanding Area VII to better reflect its content. Therefore, the new Area VII title reads: "Communicate, Promote, and Advocate for Health, Health Education/Promotion, and the Profession." Whereas in the HEJA 2010 Model the title for Area VII read: "Communicate and Advocate for Health and Health Education." The decision to add the word promotion was not a change made lightly. In fact, the HESPA 2015-TF found this decision required additional input from others in the profession. The HESPA 2015-TF implemented an online data collection initiative to elicit reactions regarding the incorporation of the concept of health promotion with the help of volunteers who participated in the study, including telephone interviewees and independent review panelists. The NCHEC Board of Commissioners and SOPHE Board of Trustees also have provided feedback. Based on the results from this survey, approximately 75% of the respondents supported adding the word "promotion," and so the term was added to the titles of each of the Seven Areas of Responsibility. Table 5.1 provides a listing of the Areas of Responsibility from the initial delineation of the role through HESPA 2015.

Section V: Changes in the Area of Responsibility: Competencies and Sub-competencies of Health Education Specialists from 1985 to 2015

Table 5.1

Comparison of Areas of Responsibility (1985 – 2015)

Entry-Level Framework (1985)	Graduate-Level Framework (1999)	CUP Model (2006)	HEJA Model (2010)	HESPA Model (2015)
I. Assessing individual and community needs for health education	I. Assessing individual and community needs for health education	I. Assess individual and community needs for education	I. Assess needs, assets, and capacity for health education	I. Assess needs, resources, and capacity for health education/promotion
II. Planning effective health education programs	II. Planning effective health education programs	II. Plan health education strategies, interventions, and programs	II. Plan health education	II. Plan health education/promotion
III. Implementing health education programs	III. Implementing health education programs	III. Implement health education strategies, interventions, and programs	III. Implement health education	III. Implement health education/promotion
IV. Evaluating effectiveness of health education programs	IV. Evaluating effectiveness of health education programs	IV. Conduct evaluation and research related to health education	IV. Conduct evaluation and research related to health education	IV. Conduct evaluation and research related to health education/promotion
V. Coordinating provision of health education services	V. Coordinating provision of health education services	V. Administer health education strategies, interventions, and programs	V. Administer and manage health education	V. Administer and manage health education/promotion
VI. Acting as a resource person in health education	VI. Acting as a resource person in health education	VI. Serve as a health education resource person	VI. Serve as a health education resource person	VI. Serve as a health education/promotion resource person
VII. Communicating health and health education needs, concerns, and resources	VII. Communicating health and health education needs, concerns, and resources	VII. Communicate and advocate for health and health education	VII. Communicate and advocate for health and health education	VII. Communicate, promote, and advocate for health, health education/ promotion, and the profession
	VIII. Applying appropriate research principles and techniques in health education			
	IX. Administering health Education programs			
	X. Advancing the profession of health education			

Note. *Adapted from Overview of the National Health Educator Competencies Updated Project, 1998-2004* by Gilmore et al. (2005), and National Commission for Health Education Credentialing, Inc., Society for Public Health Education, and American Association for Health Education. (2010). *A Competency-Based Framework for Health Education Specialists – 2010.* Whitehall, PA: National Commission for Health Education Credentialing, Inc.

Section V: Changes in the Area of Responsibility: Competencies and Sub-competencies of Health Education Specialists from 1985 to 2015

Competencies and Sub-competencies

Like the Areas of Responsibility, the Competencies and Sub-competencies also have changed over the years. In Table 5.2, the number of Competencies and Sub-competencies in HEJA 2010 Model is compared to the HESPSA 2015 Model. Table 5.2 reveals the increase in the total number of Sub-competencies from 223 in the HEJA 2010 Model to 258 in the HESPA 2015 Model. The Sub-competencies also differ according to their levels of practice within the HEJA 2010 and HESPA 2015 Models. Of the 223 Sub-competencies in the HEJA 2010 Model, 162 (72.6%) were validated at the entry-level, 42 (18.8%) at the advanced 1-level, and 19 (8.5%) at the advanced 2-level. Of the 258 Sub-competencies in the HESPA 2015 Model, 141 (54.7%) were validated at the entry-level, 76 (29.5%) were validated at the advanced 1-level, and 41 (15.9%) were validated at the advanced 2-level. The expanded number of Sub-competencies in the Areas of Responsibility helps to further delineate the Competencies being practiced by health education specialists.

The Sub-competencies of the HESPA 2015 Model that are practiced exclusively at the advanced 2-level fall into two Areas of Responsibility: *Area of Responsibility IV Conduct Evaluation and Research Related to Health Education/Promotion* and *Area of Responsibility VII Communicate, Promote, and Advocate for Health, Health Education/Promotion, and the Profession*. The Sub-competencies validated at the advanced 2-level of practice primarily relate to planning research, collecting and analyzing data, working with data collection instruments, interpreting and disseminating research findings, and mentoring less experienced health education specialists. The Sub-competencies practiced by advanced 1-level health education specialists, but not entry-level health education specialists, predominantly relate to administrative and management roles.

The three distinct levels of practice initially established through the CUP study were reverified in both the HEJA 2010 Model and the HESPA 2015 Model. These levels consist of entry-, advanced 1-, and advanced 2-levels. Consistent with earlier practice analyses, these practice levels are hierarchical in the HESPA 2015 Model. The Sub-competencies in the advanced 1-level include *generic* Sub-competencies at the entry-level and Sub-competencies specific to the advanced 1-level practice. The Sub-competencies in the advanced 2-level include generic (entry-level) Sub-competencies, advanced 1-level Sub-competencies, and an additional set of Sub-competencies specific to advanced 2-level practice.

Section V: Changes in the Area of Responsibility: Competencies and Sub-competencies of Health Education Specialists from 1985 to 2015

Table 5.2

Competencies and Sub-competencies at Each Level of Practice between the HEJA 2010 Model and the HESPA 2015 Model

Area of Responsibilities	Competencies		Total Sub-competencies		Entry-level		Advanced 1-level		Advanced 2-level	
	HEJA	HESPA	HEJA	HESPA	HEJA	HESPA	HEJA	HESPA	HEJA	HESPA
Area I	7	7	40	33	34	30	2	3	4	0
Area II	5	5	29	34	21	28	6	6	2	0
Area III	3	4	20	29	15	21	5	8	0	0
Area IV	5	7	34	57	25	9	0	10	9	38
Area V	5	6	37	51	19	18	18	33	0	0
Area VI	3	3	23	16	12	5	11	11	0	0
Area VII	6	4	40	38	36	30	0	5	4	3
Total	34	36	223	258	162	141	42	76	19	41

Area of Responsibility I: Assess Needs, Resources, and Capacity for Health Education/Promotion.

In Area of Responsibility I, there is no change in the number of Competencies from the HEJA 2010 Model to HESPA 2015 Model. Both have seven; however, there are minor wording changes in the revised Competencies. The most noticeable change is the wording of *Competency 1.3*, which changed from: *Collect quantitative and/or qualitative data related to health* changing to *Collect primary data to determine needs*. This change was made because it was assumed primary data could include both quantitative and qualitative data. The change in the wording of *Competency 1.3* makes it necessary to shift the Sub-competencies for secondary data collection to *Competency 1.2 Access existing information and data related to health.* The total number of Sub-competencies in *Area of Responsibility I* decreased from 40 in the HEJA 2010 Model to 33 in the HESPA 2015 Model. This change primarily resulted from the combination of multiple Sub-competencies from HEJA 2010 Model in the HESPA 2015 Model. For example, in the HEJA 2010 Model Competencies 1.4.1 and 1.4.2 read: *Identify factors that influence health behavior* and *Analyze factors that influence health behavior.* In the HESPA 2015 Model these Competencies were combined to form *Sub-competency 1.4.1 Identify and analyze factors that influence health behavior.*

Section V: Changes in the Area of Responsibility: Competencies and Sub-competencies of Health Education Specialists from 1985 to 2015

Area of Responsibility II: Plan Health Education/Promotion

In Area of Responsibility II, the number of Competencies remained the same at five, while the number of Sub-competencies increased from 29 in the HEJA 2010 Model to 34 in the HESPA 2015 Model. Most of the additional Sub-competencies were added to *Competencies 2.3* and *2.4*. Although the title of *Competency 2.3 Select or Design strategies/interventions* stayed the same, the additional Sub-competencies can be attributed to a further delineation of the Competency. Therefore, the HESPA 2015 Model *Competency 2.3* includes new Sub-competencies that address "applying evidence-based principles," "adapting existing strategies/interventions," "piloting testing strategies/interventions," and "refining strategies/interventions based on pilot feedback." *Competency 2.4* changed to include both a new title and additional Sub-competencies. The new title reads: *Competency 2.4 Develop a plan for the delivery of health education/promotion*. The additional Sub-competencies under *Competency 2.4* highlight the increasing number of tasks necessary to plan for implementation beyond developing a scope and sequence.

Area of Responsibility III: Implement Health Education/Promotion

Area of Responsibility III incorporates two significant changes: the addition of a new Competency and a shift in the sequence of the other Competencies to match a common flow of tasks carried out by health education specialists when implementing health education/promotion plans. The newly added Competency, *Competency 3.1 Coordinate logistics necessary to implement a plan*, includes six Sub-competencies to be addressed before implementation takes place. The remaining three Competencies in this Area of Responsibility are very similar to those found in the HEJA-2010 Model, and focus on training, implementing, and monitoring health education/promotion plans. The biggest difference between the HEJA-2010 and HESPA 2015 Models is the order in which Competencies appear. Training Competencies appear before rather than after implementing and monitoring Competencies. The addition of a fourth Competency, as well as new Sub-competencies under the remaining three Competencies, increased the total number of Sub-competencies in the Area III to 29

Area of Responsibility IV: Conduct Evaluation and Research Related to Health Education/Promotion

Area of Responsibility IV expanded from five Competencies and 34 Sub-competencies in the HEJA 2010 Model to seven Competencies and 57 Sub-competencies in HESPA 2015 Model. Two of the HEJA 2010 Model Competencies expanded to separate key concepts (i.e., *Competency 4.1 Develop Evaluation/Research Plan* and *Competency 4.3 Collect and analyze evaluation/research data*, and four new Competencies in the HESPA 2015 Model. In the HESPA 2015 Model, more emphasis is placed on developing an evaluation and research plan by separating the process into two Competencies: *Competency 4.1 Develop*

Section V: Changes in the Area of Responsibility: Competencies and Sub-competencies of Health Education Specialists from 1985 to 2015

an evaluation plan for health education/promotion and *Competency 4.2 Develop a research plan for health education/promotion*. This, in turn, increased the number of Sub-competencies associated with the process by 10. These additional components better distinguish between the skills and knowledge needed for the separate processes of evaluation and research. A split in the HEJA 2010 Model *Competency 4.3 Collect and analyze evaluation/research data* achieved similar results. This split distinguishes HESPA 2015 Model Competencies: *Competency 4.4 Collect and manage data* and *Competency 4.5 Analyze data*. This separation accounts for an increase of five Sub-competencies. The other three Competencies found in Area of Responsibility IV of the HEJA 2010 Model remained the same, with the exception of a new numbering sequence in both the Competencies and the Sub-competencies that followed. In the HESPA 2015 Model, the percentage of the Sub-competencies validated at an advanced-level of practice also changed in this Area of Responsibility. In the HEJA 2010 Model, 26.5% (9 of 34) of the Sub-competencies are validated at an advanced-level, while in the HESPA 2015 Model 84.2% (48 of 57) were validated at an advanced-level of practice. Of the 48 advanced-level Sub-competencies, 38 (79.2%) of them were validated at the advanced 2-level.

Area of Responsibility V: Administer and Manage Health Education/Promotion

Area of Responsibility V expanded from five Competencies and 37 Sub-competencies in the HEJA 2010 Model to six Competencies and 51 Sub-competencies in HESPA 2015 Model. The HESPA 2015 Model retained five Competencies from the HEJA 2010 Model, but the wording and the order of presentation of these five Competencies changed slightly. Within the five Competencies, a number of Sub-competencies were added to more clearly define the skills needed by health education specialists. For example, in the HEJA 2010 Model, *Competency 5.1* was stated *Competency 5.1 Manage fiscal resources*, while the parallel Competency in the HESPA 2015 Model reads *Competency 5.1 Manage financial resources for health education/promotion programs*. The revised Competency includes 13 Sub-competencies as opposed to six Sub-competencies in the HEJA 2010 Model to more accurately describe the skills necessary for managing financial resources. In the HESPA 2015 Model, a new Competency was added to this Area of Responsibility in order to address the increasing importance of technology. This Competency, *Competency 5.2, Manage technology resources*, includes four new Sub-competencies that are not part of the HEJA 2010 Model. The percentage of the Sub-competencies validated at an advanced-level of practice increased in this Area of Responsibility. In the HEJA 2010 Model, 48.6% (18 of 37) of the Sub-competencies were validated at an advanced-level, while in the HESPA 2015 Model 64.7% (33 of 51) were validated at an advanced-level of practice. All 33 of the advanced-level Sub-competencies were validated at the advanced 1-level.

Section V: Changes in the Area of Responsibility: Competencies and Sub-competencies of Health Education Specialists from 1985 to 2015

Area of Responsibility VI: Serve as a Health Education/Promotion Resource Person

Of the Seven Areas of Responsibility, the least amount of change from the HEJA 2010 Model to the HESPA 2015 Model occurred in Area of Responsibility VI. The number of Competencies from the HEJA 2010 Model to the HESPA 2015 Model remained the same at three. However, the titles of the three Competencies incorporated minor changes, and the Sub-competencies decreased in number from 23 to 16. The most notable change in Area of Responsibility VI was in the *consultation* Sub-competency. In the HEJA 2010 Model, the majority of the training Sub-competencies were validated at the entry-level. In the HESPA 2015 Model, the word *advice* was added to *Competency 6.3*, which reads: *Provide advice and consultation on health education/promotion issues.* All of these Sub-competencies were validated at the advanced-level of practice.

Area of Responsibility VII: Communicate, Promote, and Advocate for Health, Health Education/Promotion, and the Profession

Area of Responsibility VII in the HESPA 2015 Model contains two fewer Competencies and two fewer Sub-competencies than the HEJA 2010 Model. These changes occurred in response to two major changes: (a) the Sub-competencies in *Competency 7.1* of the HEJA 2010 Model were moved to other Competencies, and (b) *Competencies 7.2* and *7.3* from the HEJA Model 2010 were combined to form a single Competency in HESPA 2015 Model because their content overlap. The new Competency in the HESPA 2015 Model is *Competency 7.1 Identify, develop, and deliver messages using a variety of communication strategies, methods, and techniques.* Although the majority (78.9%) of the 38 Sub-competencies in this Area of Responsibility are entry-level Sub-competencies, twice as many Sub-competencies (8 as opposed to 4) were validated at an advanced-level in the HESPA 2015 study.

This page was
intentionally left blank

Section VI: Core Knowledge Items

The ability to effectively perform a professional Competency is dependent in part on the mastery of relevant knowledge. However, clearly defining knowledge bases that are essential and generic to a Competency-based framework can be a challenge. The process of integrating a knowledge-based survey into a health education/promotion job analysis was first completed during HEJA 2010. This process was undertaken to identify and verify core knowledge items for use in various aspects of professional preparation, credentialing, and professional development. A similar process was repeated with HESPA 2015 because the verified core knowledge items have been useful to those creating professional preparation programs, continuing education opportunities, and to those responsible for creating the certification examinations.

As indicated in Section II, the knowledge list developed in the HEJA 2010 Model was used as the foundation for the knowledge list created for the HESPA 2015 Model. The older list was augmented with emerging areas of knowledge and organized into 10 conceptually related topic areas by the HESPA 2015-TF and HESPA 2015 -SC. The resulting 132 knowledge items were included in the HESPA survey. The same 4-point scale used to rate the Sub-competencies was adopted for rating the knowledge statements. Participants were asked to answer the following question: *How frequently did you use the knowledge in your job as a health education specialist during the past 12 months?* Respondents the were asked to answer with one of the following: *Not at all, occasionally (less than once a month), frequently (at least once each month, very frequently (at least once each week).* At least 50% of participants used 131 of the 132 items included in the survey, and these items have been included in the list provided on the following pages.

A volunteer team of health education specialists with expertise in Competency development and credentialing reviewed each knowledge item and assigned it to at least one of the Seven Areas of Responsibility in the HESPA 2015 Model. Table 6.1 contains the knowledge items (n=131) listed by conceptually related topics with the specific Area(s) to which each item was assigned designated by a * in the table. This table can be used by university faculty who teach courses to which one or more of the Seven Areas of Responsibility have been assigned. The course instructor should ensure that the designated knowledge is addressed in the assigned course so students will be equipped with the knowledge needed to address related Competencies. Leaders of professional development efforts can use the table in the same manner and incorporate the knowledge into professional development events. Students and individual practitioners can also use the table as a guide for understanding and addressing needed knowledge bases when preparing for certification examinations or in self-guided professional development efforts.

These 131 verified knowledge items are not considered an exhaustive representation of all essential core knowledge, and some items on the list may overlap in some ways. Yet, each item on the list was empirically verified as essential to the work of at least 50% of the health education specialists who participated in the study. As such, the list of core knowledge may serve as a useful first step in establishing core knowledge items that are essential to the Competency-based framework for health education specialists. Additional research in future practice analyses is recommended to further explore and develop a broad knowledge base that is both generic and essential to the practice of health education specialists.

Section VI: Core Knowledge Items

Table 6.1
Validated Knowledge Items by Topic and Area of Responsibility

	VALIDATED KNOWLEDGE ITEM	Area I	Area II	Area III	Area IV	Area V	Area VI	Area VII
	Knowledge of: HEALTH EDUCATION PROFESSION							
001	Health education practice, history, laws, rules, regulations (for example, Privacy, HIPPA)	*	*		*	*	*	*
002	Health education, definitions							*
003	Health education programs, elements of	*	*	*	*	*		*
004	Health education specialist, role and responsibilities						*	*
005	Health education, credentialing							*
006	Health education, professional associations	*						*
007	Health education, standards	*	*	*	*	*	*	*
008	Health promotion		*	*	*		*	*
009	School health education, student standards (for example, national health education standards)		*					
010	School health education, professional preparation and licensure							*
011	Workplace health promotion, principles and methods	*	*	*	*			
012	Community/public health education, professional preparation						*	*
013	Community/public health education, accreditation							*
014	Professional development, principles and practices							
	Knowledge of: THEORIES, TECHNIQUES							
015	Education theories		*	*			*	
016	Andragogy, principles and methods	*	*	*	*		*	*
017	Pedagogy, principles and methods	*	*	*	*		*	
018	Health literacy, linguistics, principles and practices	*	*	*	*		*	*
019	Health numeracy, principles and practices		*	*	*		*	*
020	Curriculum development		*	*	*			
021	Training, principles and methods	*	*	*	*	*	*	
022	Resources, for education (selection, use, and evaluation)	*	*	*	*	*	*	*
023	Cultural/diversity competence, principles and practices	*	*	*	*	*	*	*

Section VI: Core Knowledge Items

	VALIDATED KNOWLEDGE ITEM	Area I	Area II	Area III	Area IV	Area V	Area VI	Area VII
024	Evidence-based practice	*	*	*	*	*	*	*
025	Logic models	*	*	*			*	
026	Health education theories and models	*	*	*	*		*	
027	Behavior change, principles, and methods	*	*	*				
028	Organization change, theory		*					
029	Health coaching, principles and methods					*		
030	Leadership, principles and practices	*				*		*
031	Group facilitation, principles and methods		*		*	*		*
032	Classroom management, principles and methods			*				
033	Mentoring, principles and methods					*		
034	Meetings, planning and facilitating		*	*		*	*	
035	Strategic planning, principles and methods		*		*			
036	Program implementation, principles and practices	*		*				
037	Program participation	*	*	*			*	
038	Program planning, models	*	*	*	*	*		
039	Program planning, principles and practices		*	*	*	*		*
040	Health in all policies, principles and practices	*	*	*		*	*	*
041	Social justice		*	*	*	*	*	*
042	Systems theory (including socio-ecological approach)	*	*	*	*		*	
043	Technology, delivering health education		*		*	*	*	*
044	Technology, non-educational use in practice		*	*			*	*
045	Technical assistance, methods		*	*		*	*	
	Knowledge of: ETHICS							
046	Ethics, principles and practices	*	*	*		*	*	*
047	Ethics, professional code of	*	*	*	*	*	*	*
	Knowledge of: CAPACITY, COMMUNITY BUILDING							
048	Capacity building, principles and methods	*				*	*	*
049	Coalitions, principles and practices		*	*		*	*	*

Section VI: Core Knowledge Items

	VALIDATED KNOWLEDGE ITEM	Area I	Area II	Area III	Area IV	Area V	Area VI	Area VII
050	Collaboration, principles and methods	*	*			*	*	*
051	Community building, principles and methods		*	*			*	*
052	Community organizing, principles, methods, theories and models		*	*			*	*
	Knowledge of: SYSTEMS							
053	Health care, US system		*			*	*	
054	Public health, US system		*			*	*	
055	Public health, non-US systems		*			*	*	
056	Health care financing					*	*	*
057	Education, US system		*			*	*	*
058	Electronic health/medical records, principles, laws, ethics	*			*			
059	Information technology, database management	*			*	*	*	
060	Information technology, informatics	*	*		*	*	*	
061	Health information security, principles (for example, HIPAA)				*	*		
062	Nonprofit boards, governance, laws, practice, and by-laws relevant to work of health education specialties	*	*	*	*	*	*	*
	Knowledge of: RESEARCH, EVALUATION, DATA COLLECTION							
063	Assessment, assets, principles and methods	*			*	*	*	
064	Assessment, health impact, principles and methods	*			*			
065	Assessment, needs, principles and methods	*						
066	Data, types of (for example, primary, secondary, qualitative, quantitative)	*			*	*	*	
067	Data characteristics (reliability, validity, fairness, unbiased)	*			*			
068	Data collection, methods	*			*	*	*	
069	Data collection, instrumentation	*			*			
070	Data analyses, qualitative procedures	*			*		*	

Section VI: Core Knowledge Items

	VALIDATED KNOWLEDGE ITEM	Area I	Area II	Area III	Area IV	Area V	Area VI	Area VII
071	Data analyses, quantitative procedures	*			*		*	
072	Statistics, descriptive	*			*	*	*	
073	Statistics, inferential	*			*		*	
074	Measurement, levels of	*			*			
075	Data, methods of reporting (for example, graphs, charts, tables, narrative)	*	*		*			
076	Databases (health data), identification, evaluation of appropriateness, and use	*			*		*	
077	Databases (literature), identification, evaluation of relevance, and use	*			*			
078	Epidemiology, principles and methods	*			*		*	
079	Evaluation, economic (for example, cost analyses, return on investment, cost/benefit issues)				*	*		
080	Evaluation, types (for example, methods, impact, outcome, formative, summative)		*		*	*	*	
081	Evaluation, models		*		*			
082	Evaluation, program	*	*		*	*		
083	Health indicators (leading health indicators)	*	*					
084	Health risk assessment/appraisal, principles and methods	*			*			
085	Professional literature, identification and use				*	*		*
086	Research, design, methods, and reporting				*			
087	Research, primary and secondary				*			
088	Research, participatory	*			*			
089	Sampling, principles and methods	*			*			
090	Pilot testing, principles and practices	*	*	*	*			*
091	Institutional Review Board (IRB), methods	*			*			
092	Quality improvement, principles and methods				*			

Section VI: Core Knowledge Items

	VALIDATED KNOWLEDGE ITEM	Area I	Area II	Area III	Area IV	Area V	Area VI	Area VII
	Knowledge of: MANAGEMENT, BUDGET, ADMINISTRATION, HUMAN RESOURCES							
093	Budgets, development and forecasting							
094	Fiscal management (for example, how a budget is implemented and kept on track, accounting, audit standards)					*		
095	Contracts, (including MOUs, MOAs) creation, negotiation, and execution					*		
096	Fund raising, principles and methods, legal issues		*			*		
097	Grants identification, proposal writing and management		*			*		
098	Grants, writing requests for proposals and reviewing applications					*		
099	Management, theory, principles and practices					*		
100	Management, para-professionals (for example, community health workers, peer counselors, patient navigators, health coach)					*		
101	Management, personnel (supervision, assessment, development)		*			*		
102	Management, volunteer recruitment, retention, supervision, and evaluation		*			*		
103	Stakeholders, identification and relationship management	*	*		*	*		*
104	Conflict resolution methods		*	*		*		
105	Planning tools (for example, timelines, Gantt charts)		*	*			*	
	Knowledge of: COMMUNICATION							
106	Communication, principles, methods, and theories	*	*	*			*	*
107	Communication, social media principles and methods		*	*				*
108	Communication, public speaking				*	*	*	*
109	Health communication models		*					
110	Marketing, principles and methods		*			*		
111	Media literacy							*

Section VI: Core Knowledge Items

	VALIDATED KNOWLEDGE ITEM	Area I	Area II	Area III	Area IV	Area V	Area VI	Area VII
112	Media relations, principles					*		*
113	Public relations		*			*	*	*
114	Social marketing		*	*				*
115	Social media		*	*				*
	Knowledge of: ADVOCACY							
116	Advocacy, principles and methods		*			*		*
117	Policy analysis and development, principles and practices							*
118	Administrative and legislative bodies and political structure							*
119	Media advocacy							*
	Knowledge of: OTHER							
120	Consulting, principles and practices						*	
121	Emergency preparedness						*	*
122	Environmental health	*					*	*
123	Health and disease, biopsychosocial model	*	*				*	
124	Health and injury (intentional/unintentional)						*	
125	Health disparities, determinants, identification, and approaches	*	*				*	*
126	Health organizations/agencies (nonprofessional)		*			*		*
127	Health, determinants of	*	*				*	
128	Health, dimensions of (for example, mental, social, physical, spiritual)	*	*				*	
129	Health, global issues						*	*
130	Prevention, levels of (primary, secondary, tertiary)							
131	Wellness/well-being	*					*	*

Note. Area I-Assess Needs, Resources, and Capacity for health Education/Promotion; Area II-Plan Health Education/Promotion; Area III-Implement Health Education/Promotion; Area IV-Conduct Evaluation and Research Related to Health Education/Promotion; Area V-Administer and Manage Health Education/Promotion; Area VI-Serve as a Health Education Promotion Resource Person; Area VII-Communicate, Promote and Advocate for Health, Health Education/Promotion, and the Profession. Knowledge item(s) link(s) to specific Area(s) of Responsibility are indicated by an asterisk (*)

This page was
intentionally left blank

REFERENCES

Airhihenbuwa, C. O., Cottrell, R. R., Adeyanju, M., Auld, M. E., Lysoby, L., & Smith, B. J. (2005). The National Health Educator Competencies Update Project: Celebrating a milestone and recommending next steps to the profession. *Health Education & Behavior, 32*(6), 722-724.

Allegrante, J. P., Airhihenbuwa, C. O., Auld, M. E., Birch, D. B., Roe, K. M., & Smith, B. J. (2004). Toward a unified system of accreditation for professional preparation in health education: Final report of the National Task Force on Accreditation in Health Education. *Health Education & Behavior, 31*(6), 1-16.

Allegrante, J. P., Barry, M. M., Airhihenbuwa, C. O., Auld, M. E., Collins, J. L., Lamarre, M. C., & et al. on behalf of the Galway Consensus Conference. (2009). Domains of core competency, standards, and quality assurance for building global capacity in health promotion: The Galway consensus conference statement. *Health Education & Behavior, 36*(3), 476-82.

Allegrante, J. P., Barry, M. M., Auld, M. E., & Lamarre, M. C. (2012). Galway revisited: Tracking global progress in core competencies and quality assurance for health education and health promotion. *Health Education & Behavior, 39*(6), 643-647.

American Association for Health Education, National Commission for Health Education Credentialing, Inc., & Society for Public Health Education. (1999). *A competency-based framework for graduate-level health educators.* Allentown, PA: Author.

American Educational Research Association, American Psychological Association, and National Council on Measurement in Education. (2014). *The standards for educational and psychological testing.* Washington, DC: American Educational Research Association.

Cleary, H. P. (1995). *The credentialing of health educators: An historical account, 1970-1990.* Allentown, PA: National Commission for Health Education Credentialing, Inc.

Cottrell, R. R., Auld, M. E., Birch, D. A., Taub, A., King, L. R., & Allegrante, J. P. (2012). Progress and directions in professional credentialing for health education in the United States. *Health Education & Behavior, 39*(6), 681-694.

Council for the Accreditation of Educator Preparation (CAEP). (2015). *History.* Retrieved from http://caepnet.org/about/history/

Council on Education for Public Health. (2005). *Accreditation criteria for public health programs.* Retrieved from http://ceph.org/criteria-procedures/

Dennis, D. L., & Mahoney, B. S. (2008). The CHES examination: Standards and statistical information. *The CHES Bulletin, 19*(1), 11.

Doyle, E. I., Caro, C. M., Lysoby, L., Auld, M. E., Smith, B., & Muenzen, P. (2012). The National Health Educator Job Analysis 2010: Process and outcomes. *Health Education & Behavior, 39*(3), 695-708.

Figueroa, J. L., Birch, D. A., King, L. R., & Cottrell, R. R. (2015). CEPH accreditation of stand-alone baccalaureate programs: A preliminary mapping exercise. *Health Promotion Practice, 16*(1), 115-121.

References

Gilmore, G. D., Olsen, L. K., Taub, A., & Connell, D. (2005). Overview of the national health educator competencies update project 1998-2004. *Health Education & Behavior, 32*(6), 725-737.

Hambleton, R. J., & Rogers, H. K. (1986). Technical advances in credentialing examinations, *Evaluation and the Health Professions, 9*(2), 205-229.

Institute for Credentialing Excellence (ICE). (2009). *Standards.* Retrieved from: http://www.credentialingexcellence.org/PublicationsandResources/Publications/Standards/tabid/390/Default.aspx

Joint Committee on Health Education and Promotion Terminology. (2012). Report of the 2011 joint committee on health education and promotion terminology. *American Journal of Health Education, 43*(2), SA, S1-S19.

Livingood, W. C., & Auld, M. E. (2001). The credentialing of a population-based profession: Lessons learned from health education certification. *Journal of Public Health Management and Practice, 7*(4), 38-45.

National Commission for Certifying Agencies. (2005). *Application for certification program accreditation.* Washington, DC: Author.

National Commission for Health Education Credentialing, Inc. (1985). *A framework for the development of competency-based curricula for entry-level health educators.* New York, NY: Author.

National Commission for Health Education Credentialing, Inc. (1996). *A competency-based framework for professional development of certified health education specialists.* Allentown, PA: Author.

National Commission for Health Education Credentialing, Inc., Society for Public Health Education, & American Association for Health Education. (2006). *A competency-based framework for health educators - 2006.* Whitehall, PA: Author.

National Commission for Health Education Credentialing, Inc., Society for Public Health Education, & American Association for Health Education. (2010). *A competency-based framework for health education specialists - 2010.* Whitehall, PA: Author.

National Commission for Health Education Credentialing, Inc., & Society for Public Health Education. (2014). Health *Education Specialist Practice Analysis 2015 (HESPA - 2015) Recommendations to the profession.* (PDF document) Retrieved from http://www.nchec.org/_files/_items/nch-mr-tab3-238/docs/executive%20summary.pdf. Whitehall, PA: Author.

National Commission for Health Education Credentialing, Inc. (2007). *The health education specialist: A study guide for professional competence* (5th ed.). Whitehall, PA: Author.

National Commission for Health Education Credentialing, Inc. (2008). *CHES exam receives "Gold Standard" NCCA accreditation.* Retrieved from http://www.nchec.org/news/what/#BM_NCH-MR-TAB2-30

References

National Commission for Health Education Credentialing, Inc. (2009). *NCHEC Board of Commissioners pass policy statement regarding the advance credential.* (PDF document) Retrieved from http://www.nchec.org/_files/_items/nch-mr-tab2-163/docs/mches%20press%20release%20%205-29-09.pdf

National Council for the Accreditation of Teacher Education. (2014). *Council for the Accreditation of Educator Preparation (CAEP).* Retrieved from www.ncate.org

Office of Management and Budget. (2000). *Standard occupational classification manual, 2000.* Washington, DC: U.S. Government Printing Office.

Professional Examination Service (1995). *Guidelines for the development, use, and evaluation of licensure and certification programs.* New York, NY: Author.

Raymond, M. R. (2002). A practical guide to practice analysis for credentialing examinations. *Educational Measurement: Issues and Practice, 21*(3), 25-37.

Society for Public Health Education. (2013). *The Affordable Care Act: Opportunities and challenges for health education specialists* (PDF Document). Retrieved from http://www.sophe.org/Sophe/PDF/ACA-Opportunities-and-Challenges-for-Health-Educators-FINAL.pdf

Society for Public Health Education, & American Association for Health Education (1997). *Standards for the preparation of graduate-level health educators.* Washington, DC: Author.

Society for Public Health Education, & American Association for Health Education. (2007). *SOPHE/AAHE baccalaureate program approval committee manual: Criteria, process, & procedures for quality assurance in community health education.* Washington, DC: Author.

Taub, A., Birch, D. A., Auld, M. E., Lysoby, L., & Rasar King, L. (2009). Strengthening quality assurance in health education: Recent milestones and future directions. *Health Promotion Practice, 10*(2), 192-200.

United States Department of Health, Education and Welfare, Health Resources Administration, Bureau of Health Manpower. (1978). *Preparation and practice of community, patient, and school health educators: Proceedings of the workshop on commonalities and differences.* Washington, DC: Division of Allied Health Professions.

United States Department of Labor, Bureau of Labor Statistics. (2014). *Health educators and community health workers.* Retrieved from http://www.bls.gov/ooh/community-and-social-service/health-educators.htm

Wilkinson, L., & Task Force on Statistical Inference. (1999). Statistical methods in psychology journals: Guidelines and explanations. *American Psychologist, 54*(8), 594-604.

This page was
intentionally left blank

APPENDIX A: GLOSSARY

The glossary is presented to explain terms used in this document. These definitions are not all inclusive, but are intended to convey the meaning of terms within the context of this document.

Advanced 1-level – The practice level of a health education specialist with a minimum of a baccalaureate degree with professional preparation in the field of health education plus various combinations of degree (baccalaureate or master's) and years of experience.

Advanced 2-level – The practice level of a health education specialist with a minimum of a doctoral degree in the field of health education, irrespective of years of experience.

Area of Responsibility – One of the major categories of performance expectations of a proficient health education practitioner. The Areas of Responsibility define the scope of practice (SOPHE & AAHE, 1997).

Certified Health Education Specialist (CHES) – "An individual who has met required academic preparation qualifications, successfully passed a competency-based examination administered by the National Commission for Health Education Credentialing, Inc., and who satisfies the continuing education requirement to maintain the national credential" (Joint Committee on Health Education and Promotion Terminology, 2012, p. S8).

Master Certified Health Education Specialist (MCHES) – "An advanced-level practitioner who has met required academic preparation qualifications, worked in the field for a minimum of five years, has successfully passed a competency-based assessment administered by the National Commission for Health Education Credentialing, Inc., and who satisfies the continuing education requirement to maintain the national credential" (Joint Committee on Health Education and Promotion Terminology, 2012, p. S8-S9).

Credentialing – An umbrella term for the process by which an entity, authorized and qualified to do so, grants formal recognition (i.e., accreditation, licensure, registration, certification) to or records the recognition status of individuals, organizations, institutions, programs, processes, services, or products that meet predetermined and standardized criteria (ICE, 2005).

Coalition – An alliance, often temporary, that allows two or more groups or organizations to promote a common cause (AAHE, NCHEC, & SOPHE, 1999).

Competency – A broadly defined skill or ability necessary for successful performance as a health education specialist.

Entry-level – The practice level of a health education specialist with a minimum of a baccalaureate degree with professional preparation in the field of health education.

Health education – "Any combination of planned learning experiences using evidence-based practices and/or sound theories that provide the opportunity to acquire knowledge, attitudes, and skills needed to adopt and maintain healthy behaviors" (Joint Committee on Health Education and Promotion Terminology, 2012, p. S12).

Health education profession – "A profession that uses evidence-based practice, and behavioral and organizational change principles to develop, plan, implement, and evaluate interventions that enable individuals, groups, and communities to achieve personal, environmental, and societal health" (Joint Committee on Health Education and Promotion Terminology, 2012, p. S12).

Appendix A: Glossary

Health education specialist – "An individual who has met, at a minimum, baccalaureate-level required academic preparation qualifications, who serves in a variety of roles, and is able to use appropriate educational strategies and methods to facilitate the development of policies, procedures, interventions, and systems conducive to the health of individuals, groups, and communities" (Joint Committee on Health Education and Promotion Terminology, 2012, p. S13).

Health literacy – "The degree to which individuals have the capacity to obtain, interpret, and understand basic health information and services and the competence to make appropriate health decisions" (Joint Committee on Health Education and Promotion Terminology, 2012, p. S13).

Health promotion – "Any combination of educational, political, environmental, regulatory, or organizational mechanisms that support actions and conditions of living that are conducive to the health of individuals, groups, and communities" (Joint Committee on Health Education and Promotion Terminology, 2012, p. S14).

Professional development – "Education and training to maintain and enhance one's competence in health education following a previously attained level of professional preparation" (Joint Committee on Health Education and Promotion Terminology, 2012, p. 14).

Professional preparation – "An undergraduate or graduate course of study based on the areas of responsibility, competencies, and sub-competencies for health education offered through an accredited college or university, that is designed to prepare individuals to practice competently in health education" (Joint Committee on Health Education and Promotion Terminology, 2012, p. 14).

Standard – The predetermined level of performance at which a criterion will be considered met. If a desired condition or characteristic (e.g., curricular content that assures development of specific health education Competencies) is the criterion, the standard then expresses the minimum acceptable content that will satisfy the expectation (AAHE, NCHEC, & SOPHE, 1999).

Sub-competency – Cluster of simpler but essential related skills or abilities within a Competency.

Appendix B: Comparison of the Competencies and Sub-competencies of the HEJA 2010 Model and the HESPA 2015 Model

The HESPA 2015 Model contains most of the Competencies and Sub-competencies of the HEJA 2010 Model, along with some additional components that reflect the contemporary practice of health education specialists at the entry-, advanced 1-, and advanced 2- levels. To adopt the HESPA 2015 Model as the framework for certification, professional preparation, and professional development, health education specialists need to adapt the criteria and materials used for these three purposes. To help facilitate these adaptations, a subcommittee from the NCHEC Division Board for Certification of Health Education compared the Areas of Responsibility, Competencies, and Sub-competencies of the HEJA 2010 Model and the HESPA 2015 Model. Tables B.1 and B.2 illustrate the results of this comparison: Table B.1 starts with the HEJA 2010 Model and Table B.2 starts with the new HESPA 2015 Model. The comparison tables were completed with the intent to direct users to similar or related Competencies and Sub-competencies that may be useful in making the transition from the HEJA Model to the HESPA Model. However, the users are urged to carefully consider the wording of the Competency or Sub-competency and make their own determination if the statement(s) apply in their particular usage.

Table B.1 can be used to identify specific Competencies and Sub-competencies in the HEJA 2010 Model that were retained, re-assigned, and/or revised and integrated into a different Area of Responsibility and/or Competency in the HESPA 2015 Model. For example, the first Competency in the HEJA 2010 Model under Area of Responsibility I was *1.1 Plan Assessment Process.* Slightly different wording with similar intent appears in the HESPA 2015 Model first Competency 1.1 *Plan assessment process for health education/promotion.* The wording of the first Sub-competency in Area of Responsibility I in the HEJA 2010 Model 1.1.1 has remained exactly the same: *Identify existing and needed resources to conduct assessments.* In the HESPA 2015 Model, the Sub-competency now appears in the second position as Sub-competency 1.1.2. This Sub-competency is underlined to indicate that the wording was an exact match.

Entries in the table with similar scope and wording that do not match exactly are identified in the right hand column, but these entries are not underlined. For example, HEJA 2010 Model *Sub-competency* 1.1.2 *Identify stakeholders to participate in the assessment process* is closely aligned with HESPA 2015 Model *Sub-competency 1.1.3 Engage priority populations, partners, and stakeholders to participate in the assessment process.*

If no apparent match was found, the words "no match" appear in the right hand column. HEJA 2010 Model *Sub-competency 1.1.6 Integrate research designs, methods, and instruments into assessment plan* provides an example of a Sub-competency with no match. Though the comparison results are useful for the realignment of items on the certification exam and for adjusting curricula in professional preparation programs, the comparison was based on specific wording, not on intent of use. Users must carefully examine the intent of use of the Competency or Sub-competency when considering the information presented in Table B.1 and B.2.

Appendix B1: Comparison of the Competencies and Sub-competencies of the HEJA 2010 Model and the HESPA 2015 Model

The levels (entry, advanced 1, and advanced 2) are indicated by symbols. The entry-level Sub-competencies no symbol, the advanced 1-level ❖, and the advanced 2-level ■. As indicated in Table B.1, some Sub-competencies in the HEJA 2010 Model may now be in a different level of practice in the HESPA 2015 Model. For example, in the HEJA 2010 Model, entry-level *Sub-competency 1.1.3 Apply theories and models to develop assessment strategies* is now shown in the HESPA 2015 Model with the same wording as *Sub-competency 1.1.4* at the advanced 1-level (note ❖ symbol in the table). Users are reminded that this Model is hierarchical, meaning the advanced-levels build on the previous level. Therefore, the entry-level Competencies and Sub-competencies apply to all levels. The advanced 2-level would also include advanced 1-level Sub-competencies.

The format of Table B.2 is similar to that of Table B.1. However, Table B.2 contains the Areas of Responsibility, Competencies, and Sub-competencies of the HESPA 2015 Model. The right hand column indicates similarly worded Competencies or Sub-competencies in the HEJA 2010 Model. For some, the word "New" is listed in that column to denote that no Competency or Sub-competency containing that specific wording existed in the HEJA 2010 Model. The same caution provided for interpreting the words "no match" in Table B.1 should also be used in interpreting the word "New" in Table B.2. It should be noted that the comparison was based on specific wording, not on intent of use. It is up to users to carefully examine the intent of use of the Competency or Sub-competency when considering the information presented in Table B.1 and B.2.

The seasoned health education specialist will likely note that the HESPA 2015 Model contains most of the Competencies and Sub-competencies of the HEJA 2010 Model, along with some additional components that reflect the contemporary practice of health education specialists at the entry-, advanced 1-, and advanced 2-levels. One of the benefits of the HESPA 2015 Model is that most Sub-competencies emerged in straightforward language with one clear function that should facilitate clear interpretation and effective application of the Model.

Appendix B1: Comparison of the Competencies and Sub-competencies of the HEJA 2010 Model and the HESPA 2015 Model

Table B.1

Comparison of the HEJA 2010 Model (Old) to the HESPA 2015 Model (New)

Many of the HEJA Sub-competencies correlate to similar HESPA Sub-competencies. If the Sub-competency is worded the same in both Frameworks, it is underlined. All advanced-1 Sub-competencies are indicated by the symbol ❖, and the advanced-2 Sub-competencies are indicated by the symbol ■. "No Match" indicates no direct/similar Sub-competency.

KEY: entry level - no symbol; advanced 1 ❖; advanced 2 ■
Sub-competency worded the same in both Frameworks is underlined.

Area I: Assess Needs, Resources, and Capacity for Health Education/Promotion		
HEJA 2010 (Old) Competencies and Sub-competencies		**Corresponding HESPA (New) Competencies and Sub-competencies**
1.1	**Plan Assessment Process**	**1.1**
1.1.1	Identify existing and needed resources to conduct assessments	1.1.2
1.1.2❖	Identify stakeholders to participate in the assessment process	1.1.3
1.1.3	Apply theories and models to develop assessment strategies	1.1.4❖
1.1.4	Develop plans for data collection, analysis, and interpretation	1.3.3
1.1.5❖	Engage stakeholders to participate in the assessment process	1.1.3
1.1.6	Integrate research designs, methods, and instruments into assessment plan	No Match
1.2	**Access Existing Information and Data Related to Health**	**1.2**
1.2.1	Identify sources of data related to health	1.2.1
1.2.2	Critique sources of health information using theory and evidence from the literature	1.2.3
1.2.3	Select valid sources of information about health	1.2.6, 6.1.2
1.2.4	Identify gaps in data using theories and assessment models	1.2.4
1.2.5	Establish collaborative relationships and agreements that facilitate access to data	1.2.2❖, 5.3.3
1.2.6	Conduct searches of existing databases for specific health-related data	1.2.1

Appendix B1: Comparison of the Competencies and Sub-competencies of the HEJA 2010 Model and the HESPA 2015 Model

KEY: entry level - no symbol; advanced 1 ❖; advanced 2 ■
Sub-competency worded the same in both Frameworks is <u>underlined</u>.

Area I: Assess Needs, Resources, and Capacity for Health Education/Promotion		
HEJA 2010 (Old) Competencies and Sub-competencies		Corresponding HESPA (New) Competencies and Sub-competencies
1.3	**Collect Quantitative and/or Qualitative Data Related to Health**	1.3
1.3.1	Collect primary and/or secondary data	1.2.5
1.3.2	Integrate primary data with secondary data	No Match
1.3.3	Identify data collection instruments and methods	1.3.1, 1.3.2, 4.3.1 ■
1.3.4	Develop data collection instruments and methods	1.3.3, 4.1.8, 4.3.3 ■, 4.3.4 ❖, 4.3.5 ❖, 4.3.6 ■, 4.3.7 ■, 4.3.8 ■, 4.3.9 ■
1.3.5	Train personnel and stakeholders regarding data collection	1.3.4
1.3.6	Use data collection instruments and methods	1.3.5
1.3.7	Employ ethical standards when collecting data	1.1.5
1.4	**Examine Relationships Among Behavioral, Environmental and Genetic Factors that Enhance or Compromise Health**	1.4
1.4.1	Identify factors that influence health behaviors	1.4.1
1.4.2	Analyze factors that influence health behaviors	1.4.1
1.4.3	Identify factors that enhance or compromise health	1.4.2
1.4.4	Analyze factors that enhance or compromise health	1.4.2
1.5	**Examine Factors that Influence the Learning Process**	1.5
1.5.1	Identify factors that foster or hinder the learning process	1.5.1, 1.5.2
1.5.2 ■	Analyze factors that foster or hinder the learning process	1.5.1, 1.5.2
1.5.3	Identify factors that foster or hinder attitudes and belief	1.5.3
1.5.4	Analyze factors that foster or hinder attitudes and beliefs	1.5.3
1.5.5 ■	Identify factors that foster or hinder skill building	1.5.4
1.5.6 ❖	Analyze factors that foster or hinder skill building	1.5.4

Appendix B1: Comparison of the Competencies and Sub-competencies of the HEJA 2010 Model and the HESPA 2015 Model

KEY: entry level - no symbol; advanced 1 ❖; advanced 2 ■
Sub-competency worded the same in both Frameworks is <u>underlined</u>.

Area I: Assess Needs, Resources, and Capacity for Health Education/Promotion		
HEJA 2010 (Old) Competencies and Sub-competencies		**Corresponding HESPA (New) Competencies and Sub-competencies**
1.6	**Examine Factors that Enhance or Compromise the Process of Health Education**	1.6
1.6.1	Determine the extent of available health education programs, interventions, and policies	1.6.1, 1.6.2
1.6.2	Assess the quality of available health education programs, interventions, and policies	1.6.3
1.6.3	Identify existing and potential partners for the provision of health education	No Match
1.6.4	Assess social, environmental, and political conditions that may impact health education	1.6.4
1.6.5	Analyze the capacity for developing needed health education	1.6.5
1.6.6	Assess the need for resources to foster health education	1.7.2, 3.1.3
1.7	**Infer Needs for Health Education Based on Assessment Findings**	1.7
1.7.1	Analyze assessment findings	No Match
1.7.2 ■	Synthesize assessment findings	<u>1.7.1</u> ❖
1.7.3	Prioritize health education needs	1.7.3
1.7.4	Identify emerging health education needs	1.4.3
1.7.5	Report assessment findings	<u>1.7.5</u>
Area II: Plan Health Education/Promotion		
2.1	**Involve Priority Populations, Partners, and other Stakeholders in the Planning Process**	2.1
2.1.1	Incorporate principles of community organization	1.7.4
2.1.2	Identify priority populations and other stakeholders	1.1.1, 2.1.1
2.1.3	Communicate need for health education to priority populations and other stakeholders	2.1.2
2.1.4	Develop collaborative efforts among priority populations and other stakeholders	2.1.3
2.1.5	Elicit input from priority populations and other stakeholders	2.1.4
2.1.6	Obtain commitments from priority populations and other stakeholders	2.1.5

Appendix B1: Comparison of the Competencies and Sub-competencies of the HEJA 2010 Model and the HESPA 2015 Model

KEY: entry level - no symbol; advanced 1 ❖; advanced 2 ■
Sub-competency worded the same in both Frameworks is underlined.

Area II: Plan Health Education/Promotion		
HEJA 2010 (Old) Competencies and Sub-competencies		**Corresponding HESPA (New) Competencies and Sub-competencies**
2.2	**Develop Goals and Objectives**	**2.2**
2.2.1❖	Use assessment results to inform the planning process	No Match
2.2.2	Identify desired outcomes utilizing the needs assessment results	2.2.1
2.2.3■	Select planning model(s) for health education	<u>2.3.1</u>❖
2.2.4❖	Develop goal statements	<u>2.2.4</u>
2.2.5❖	Formulate specific, measurable, attainable, realistic, and time-sensitive objectives	2.2.5
2.2.6	Assess resources needed to achieve objectives	2.4.2❖
2.3	**Select or Design Strategies and Interventions**	**2.3**
2.3.1■	Assess efficacy of various strategies to ensure consistency with objectives	2.3.2❖, 3.4.3
2.3.2	Design theory-based strategies and interventions to achieve stated objectives	2.3.3❖, 2.3.8
2.3.3❖	Select a variety of strategies and interventions to achieve stated objectives	2.3.3❖
2.3.4	Comply with legal and ethical principles in designing strategies and interventions	2.3.11, 2.3.12
2.3.5	Apply principles of cultural competence in selecting and designing strategies and interventions	<u>2.3.4</u>, 2.3.5
2.3.6	Pilot test strategies and interventions	2.3.9❖, 2.4.10
2.4	**Develop a Scope and Sequence for the Delivery of Health Education**	**2.4**
2.4.1	Determine the range of health education needed to achieve goals and objectives	No Match
2.4.2	Select resources required to implement health education	2.4.2, 3.1.3
2.4.3	Use logic models to guide the planning process	2.4.1
2.4.4❖	Organize health education into a logical sequence	<u>2.4.3</u>
2.4.5❖	Develop a timeline for the delivery of health education	<u>2.4.4</u>
2.4.6	Analyze the opportunity for integrating health education into other programs	<u>2.4.7</u>
2.4.7	Develop a process for integrating health education into other programs	2.4.8❖

Appendix B1: Comparison of the Competencies and Sub-competencies of the HEJA 2010 Model and the HESPA 2015 Model

KEY: entry level - no symbol; advanced 1 ❖; advanced 2 ■
Sub-competency worded the same in both Frameworks is <u>underlined</u>.

Area II: Plan Health Education/Promotion		
HEJA 2010 (Old) Competencies and Sub-competencies		Corresponding HESPA (New) Competencies and Sub-competencies
2.5	**Address Factors that Affect Implementation**	2.5
2.5.1	Identify factors that foster or hinder implementation	2.5.1
2.5.2	Analyze factors that foster or hinder implementation	2.5.1
2.5.3	Use findings of pilot to refine implementation plans as needed	2.3.10❖, 2.4.10
2.5.4	Develop a conducive learning environment	2.3.6, 3.1.1
Area III: Implement Health Education/Promotion		
3.1	**Implement a Plan of Action**	3.3
3.1.1	Assess readiness for implementation	<u>3.3.3</u>
3.1.2	Collect baseline data	<u>3.3.1</u>
3.1.3	Use strategies to ensure cultural competence in implementing health education plans	3.3.4
3.1.4	Use a variety of strategies to deliver a plan of action	3.3.6, <u>3.3.7</u>
3.1.5	Promote plan of action	2.4.5, 3.3.5
3.1.6	Apply theories and models of implementation	<u>3.3.2</u>❖
3.1.7	Launch plan of action	3.3.6
3.2	**Monitor Implementation of Health Education**	3.4❖
3.2.1	Monitor progress in accordance with timeline	<u>3.4.1</u>
3.2.2	Assess progress in achieving objectives	<u>3.4.2</u>❖
3.2.3	Modify plan of action as needed	<u>3.4.4</u>❖
3.2.4	Monitor use of resources	<u>3.4.5</u>❖
3.2.5	Monitor compliance with legal and ethical principles	3.1.5, 3.1.6, 3.4.7, 3.4.8
3.3	**Train Individuals Involved in Implementation of Health Education**	3.2
3.3.1	Select training participants needed for implementation	3.2.2
3.3.2❖	Identify training needs	3.2.3❖
3.3.3❖	Develop training objectives	<u>3.2.1</u>❖

Appendix B1: Comparison of the Competencies and Sub-competencies of the HEJA 2010 Model and the HESPA 2015 Model

KEY: entry level - no symbol; advanced 1 ❖; advanced 2 ■
Sub-competency worded the same in both Frameworks is <u>underlined</u>.

Area III: Implement Health Education/Promotion		
HEJA 2010 (Old) Competencies and Sub-competencies		Corresponding HESPA (New) Competencies and Sub-competencies
3.3.4❖	Create training using best practices	3.2.4❖
3.3.5	Demonstrate a wide range of training strategies	3.2.4❖
3.3.6	Deliver training	3.2.5❖
3.3.7❖	Evaluate training	<u>3.2.7</u>❖
3.3.8❖	Use evaluation findings to plan future training	3.2.8❖
Area IV: Conduct Evaluation and Research Related to Health Education/Promotion		
4.1	Develop Evaluation/Research Plan	4.1, 4.2
4.1.1■	Create purpose statement	4.1.1❖, 4.2.1■
4.1.2■	Develop evaluation/research questions	4.1.2❖, 4.2.5■
4.1.3	Assess feasibility of conducting evaluation/research	4.1.5❖, 4.2.2■
4.1.4	Critique evaluation and research methods and findings found in the related literature	4.2.3■, 4.2.4■
4.1.5	Synthesize information found in the literature	4.2.3■, 4.2.4■
4.1.6	Assess the merits and limitations of qualitative and quantitative data collection for evaluation	4.1.6❖, 4.2.6■
4.1.7■	Assess the merits and limitations of qualitative and quantitative date collection for research	4.1.6❖, 4.2.6■
4.1.8	Identify existing data collection instruments	4.2.8■, <u>4.3.1</u>■
4.1.9	Critique existing data collection instruments for evaluation	4.3.1■, 4.3.2■
4.1.10■	Critique existing data collection instruments for research	4.3.1■, 4.3.2■
4.1.11■	Create a logic model to guide the evaluation process	<u>4.1.3</u>❖, 4.1.4❖
4.1.12	Develop data analysis plan for evaluation	4.1.9■
4.1.13■	Develop data analysis plan for research	4.2.12■
4.1.14	Apply ethical standards in developing the evaluation/research plan	4.1.10❖, 4.2.14■

Appendix B1: Comparison of the Competencies and Sub-competencies of the HEJA 2010 Model and the HESPA 2015 Model

KEY: entry level - no symbol; advanced 1 ❖; advanced 2 ■
Sub-competency worded the same in both Frameworks is <u>underlined</u>.

Area IV: Conduct Evaluation and Research Related to Health Education/Promotion		
HEJA 2010 (Old) Competencies and Sub-competencies		Corresponding HESPA (New) Competencies and Sub-competencies
4.2	**Design Instruments to Collect**	4.3
4.2.1	Identify useable questions from existing instruments	4.3.4 ❖
4.2.2	Write new items to be used in data collection for evaluation	4.3.5, 4.3.6 ■
4.2.3 ■	Write new items to be used in data collection for research	4.3.5, 4.3.6 ■
4.2.4	Establish validity of data collection instruments	<u>4.3.8</u> ■
4.2.5	Establish reliability of data collection instruments	4.3.9 ■
4.3	**Collect and Analyze Evaluation/Research Data**	4.4 ■, 4.5 ■
4.3.1	Collect data based on the evaluation/research plan	4.4.1 ■, <u>4.4.2</u> ■
4.3.2	Monitor data collection and management	4.4.3 ■, 4.4.4 ❖
4.3.3	Analyze data using inferential and/or other advanced statistical methods	4.5.4
4.3.4	Analyze data using qualitative methods	<u>4.5.2</u> ❖
4.3.5	Apply ethical standards in collecting and analyzing data	4.1.10 ❖
4.4	**Interpret Results of the Evaluation/Research**	4.6
4.4.1	Compare results to evaluation/research questions	4.6.2 ■
4.4.2	Compare results to other findings	4.6.3 ■
4.4.3	Propose possible explanations of findings	<u>4.6.4</u> ■, 4.6.7 ■
4.4.4	Identify possible limitations of findings	<u>4.6.5</u> ■, 4.6.6 ■
4.4.5	Develop recommendations based on results	<u>4.6.8</u> ■
4.5	**Apply Findings from Evaluation/Research**	4.7
4.5.1	Communicate findings to stakeholders	4.7.1, 4.7.2
4.5.2 ■	Evaluate feasibility of implementing recommendations from evaluation	4.7.3
4.5.3	Apply evaluation findings in policy analysis and program development	4.7.4
4.5.4 ■	Disseminate research findings through professional conference	4.7.5 ■

Appendix B1: Comparison of the Competencies and Sub-competencies of the HEJA 2010 Model and the HESPA 2015 Model

KEY: entry level - no symbol; advanced 1 ❖; advanced 2 ■
Sub-competency worded the same in both Frameworks is <u>underlined</u>.

Area V: Administer and Manage Health Education		
HEJA 2010 (Old) Competencies and Sub-competencies		**Corresponding HESPA (New) Competencies and Sub-competencies**
5.1	**Manage Fiscal Resources**	**5.1**
5.1.1❖	Identify fiscal and other resources	5.1.3
5.1.2❖	Prepare requests/proposals to obtain fiscal resources	5.1.4
5.1.3❖	Develop budgets to support health education efforts	5.1.5
5.1.4❖	Manage program budgets	<u>5.1.6</u>
5.1.5❖	Prepare budget reports	<u>5.1.8</u>
5.1.6❖	Demonstrate ethical behavior in managing fiscal resources	5.1.13
5.2	**Obtain Acceptance and Support for Programs**	**5.4**
5.2.1❖	Use communication strategies to obtain program support	5.4.3, 5.4.4
5.2.2❖	Facilitate cooperation among stakeholders responsible for health education	5.3.2❖, 5.3.3
5.2.3❖	Prepare reports to obtain and/or maintain program support	5.4.1, 5.4.2, 5.4.3, 5.4.4
5.2.4❖	Synthesize data for purposes of reporting	4.6.1■, 5.2.2
5.2.5	Provide support for individuals who deliver professional development opportunities	5.6.8❖
5.2.6	Explain how program goals align with organizational structure, mission and goals	2.2.3, 5.4.1
5.3	**Demonstrate Leadership**	**5.5**
5.3.1	Conduct strategic planning	<u>5.5.5</u>❖, <u>5.5.6</u>❖, <u>5.5.7</u>❖
5.3.2	Analyze an organization's culture in relationship to health education goals	5.5.2
5.3.3❖	Promote collaboration among stakeholders	5.3.2❖, 5.3.3
5.3.4	Develop strategies to reinforce or change organizational culture to achieve health education goals	5.5.3
5.3.5	Comply with existing laws and regulations	4.4.5, <u>5.5.9</u>
5.3.6	Adhere to ethical standards of the profession	<u>5.5.10</u>
5.3.7	Facilitate efforts to achieve organizational mission	2.2.3, <u>5.5.1</u>❖
5.3.8	Analyze the need for a systems approach to change	7.3.3, 7.3.4
5.3.9	Facilitate needed changes to organizational cultures	<u>5.5.4</u>❖

Appendix B1: Comparison of the Competencies and Sub-competencies of the HEJA 2010 Model and the HESPA 2015 Model

KEY: entry level - no symbol; advanced 1 ❖; advanced 2 ■
Sub-competency worded the same in both Frameworks is <u>underlined</u>.

Area V: Administer and Manage Health Education		
HEJA 2010 (Old) Competencies and Sub-competencies		Corresponding HESPA (New) Competencies and Sub-competencies
5.4	**Manage Human Resources**	5.6
5.4.1	Develop volunteer opportunities	5.6.4❖, 5.6.6❖
5.4.2	Demonstrate leadership skills in managing human resources	5.6.3❖, 5.6.14❖
5.4.3	Apply human resource policies consistent with relevant laws and regulations	<u>5.6.3</u>❖
5.4.4	Evaluate qualifications of staff and volunteers needed for programs	5.6.3❖
5.4.5	Recruit volunteers and staff	5.6.5
5.4.6	Employ conflict resolution strategies	5.6.10
5.4.7	Apply appropriate methods for team development	5.6.11
5.4.8	Model professional practices and ethical behavior	5.6.14❖
5.4.9❖	Develop strategies to enhance staff and volunteers' career development	5.6.7
5.4.10❖	Implement strategies to enhance staff and volunteers' career development	5.6.8❖
5.4.11	Evaluate performance of staff and volunteers	<u>5.6.12</u>❖
5.5	**Facilitate Partnerships in Support of Health Education**	5.5
5.5.1❖	Identify potential partner(s)	5.3.1
5.5.2❖	Assess capacity of potential partner(s) to meet program goals	5.3.1
5.5.3	Facilitate partner relationship(s)	5.3.2❖, 5.3.3, 5.3.4
5.5.4❖	Elicit feedback from partner(s)	5.3.5❖, 5.3.4
5.5.5❖	Evaluate feasibility of continuing partnership	5.3.6
Area VI: Serve as a Health Education Resource Person		
6.1	**Obtain and Disseminate Health-Related Information**	6.1
6.1.1	Assess information needs	6.1.1
6.1.2	Identify valid information resources	<u>6.1.2</u>
6.1.3	Critique resource materials for accuracy, relevance, and timeliness	6.1.2
6.1.4	Convey health-related information to priority populations	6.1.4, 6.1.5
6.1.5	Convey health-related information to key stakeholders	6.1.4, 6.1.5

Appendix B1: Comparison of the Competencies and Sub-competencies of the HEJA 2010 Model and the HESPA 2015 Model

KEY: entry level - no symbol; advanced 1 ❖; advanced 2 ■
Sub-competency worded the same in both Frameworks is <u>underlined</u>.

Area VI: Serve as a Health Education Resource Person		
HEJA 2010 (Old) Competencies and Sub-competencies		Corresponding HESPA (New) Competencies and Sub-competencies
6.2	**Provide Training**	6.2
6.2.1❖	Analyze requests for training	6.2.1❖
6.2.2❖	Prioritize requests for training	6.2.2❖
6.2.3❖	Identify priority populations	1.1.1, 2.1.1
6.2.4❖	Assess needs for training	6.2.1❖
6.2.5❖	Identify existing resources that meet training needs	6.2.3❖
6.2.6❖	Use learning theory to develop or adapt training programs	2.3.8, 3.2.4❖
6.2.7❖	Develop training plan	6.2.2❖
6.2.8❖	Implement training sessions and programs	6.2.4❖
6.2.9❖	Use a variety of resources and strategies	3.2.5❖, 6.2.4❖
6.2.10❖	Evaluate impact of training programs	3.2.7❖, 6.2.5❖
6.3	**Serve as a Health Education Consultant**	6.3
6.3.1	Assess needs for assistance	6.3.1❖
6.3.2	Prioritize requests for assistance	6.3.1❖
6.3.3	Define parameters of effective consultative relationships	6.3.2❖
6.3.4	Establish consultative relationships	6.3.2❖
6.3.5❖	Provide expert assistance	6.3.3❖
6.3.6	Facilitate collaborative efforts to achieve program goals	5.3.3❖
6.3.7❖	Evaluate the effectiveness of the expert assistance provided	6.3.4❖
6.3.8	Apply ethical principles in consultative relationships	6.3.5❖
Area VII: Communicate and Advocate for Health and Health Education		
7.1	**Assess and Prioritize Health Information and Advocacy Needs**	No Match
7.1.1	Identify current and emerging issues that may influence health and health education	5.2.4, 7.2.1
7.1.2	Access accurate resources related to identified issues	5.1.2❖
7.1.3	Analyze the impact of existing and proposed policies on health	<u>7.3.1</u>
7.1.4	Analyze factors that influence decision-makers	7.3.7❖, 7.3.8❖, 7.3.9

Appendix B1: Comparison of the Competencies and Sub-competencies of the HEJA 2010 Model and the HESPA 2015 Model

KEY: entry level - no symbol; advanced 1 ❖; advanced 2 ■
Sub-competency worded the same in both Frameworks is <u>underlined</u>.

Area VII: Communicate and Advocate for Health and Health Education		
HEJA 2010 (Old) Competencies and Sub-competencies		**Corresponding HESPA (New) Competencies and Sub-competencies**
7.2	**Identify and Develop a Variety of Communication Strategies, Methods, and Techniques**	7.1
7.2.1	Create messages using communication theories and models	<u>7.1.1</u>
7.2.2	Tailor messages to priority populations	2.3.7, <u>7.1.3</u>
7.2.3	Incorporate images to enhance messages	7.1.7
7.2.4	Select effective methods or channels for communicating to priority populations	<u>2.4.6</u>, 7.1.6, 7.1.7
7.2.5	Pilot test messages and delivery methods with priority populations	<u>7.1.4</u>❖
7.2.6	Revise messages based on pilot feedback	<u>7.1.5</u>❖
7.3	**Deliver Messages Using a Variety of Strategies, Methods, and Techniques**	7.1
7.3.1	Use techniques that empower individuals and communities to improve their health	7.1.7
7.3.2	Employ technology to communicate to priority populations	5.2.1
7.3.3	Evaluate the delivery of communication strategies, methods, and techniques	2.4.9
7.4	**Engage in Health Education Advocacy**	7.2
7.4.1	Engage stakeholders in advocacy	<u>7.2.2</u>
7.4.2	Develop an advocacy plan in compliance with local, state, and/or federal policies and procedures	<u>7.2.4</u>
7.4.3	Comply with organizational policies related to participating in advocacy	<u>7.2.8</u>
7.4.4	Communicate the impact of health and health education on organizational and socio-ecological factors	7.2.9
7.4.5	Use data to support advocacy messages	7.2.3, 7.2.5
7.4.6	Implement advocacy plans	<u>7.2.6</u>
7.4.7	Incorporate media and technology in advocacy	5.2.4, 7.2.5
7.4.8	Participate in advocacy initiatives	7.3.10
7.4.9 ■	Lead advocacy initiatives	7.2.9
7.4.10 ■	Evaluate advocacy efforts	<u>7.2.7</u>

Appendix B1: Comparison of the Competencies and Sub-competencies of the HEJA 2010 Model and the HESPA 2015 Model

KEY: entry level - no symbol; advanced 1 ❖; advanced 2 ■
Sub-competency worded the same in both Frameworks is <u>underlined</u>.

Area VII: Communicate and Advocate for Health and Health Education		
HEJA 2010 (Old) Competencies and Sub-competencies		Corresponding HESPA (New) Competencies and Sub-competencies
7.5	**Influence Policy to Promote Health**	**7.3**
7.5.1 ■	Use evaluation and research findings in policy analysis	7.3.1, 7.3.2, 7.3.5
7.5.2	Identify the significance and implications of health policy for individuals, groups, and communities	7.2.5
7.5.3	Advocate for health-related policies, regulations, laws, or rules	7.2.5, 7.3.10
7.5.4 ■	Use evidence-based research to develop policies to promote health	7.3.5, 7.3.6 ❖
7.5.5	Employ policy and media advocacy techniques to influence decision-makers	7.3.8 ❖, 7.3.9
7.6	**Promote the Health Education Profession**	**7.4**
7.6.1	Develop a personal plan for professional growth and service	7.4.8
7.6.2	Describe state-of-the-art health education practice	7.4.1
7.6.3	Explain the major responsibilities of the health education specialist in the practice of health education	7.4.1
7.6.4	Explain the role of health education associations in advancing the profession	<u>7.4.2</u>
7.6.5	Explain the benefits of participating in professional organizations	<u>7.4.3</u>, 7.4.5
7.6.6	Facilitate professional growth of self and others	7.4.4
7.6.7	Explain the history of the health education profession and its current and future implications for professional practice	<u>7.4.6</u>
7.6.8	Explain the role of credentialing in the promotion of the health education profession	7.4.7
7.6.9	Engage in professional development activities	7.4.8
7.6.10	Serve as a mentor to others	7.4.9 ■
7.6.11	Develop materials that contribute to the professional literature	7.4.10 ■
7.6.12	Engage in service to advance the health education profession	7.4.11 ■

Appendix B2: Comparison of the Competencies and Sub-competencies of the HESPA 2015 Model and the HEJA 2010 Model

Table B.2.

Comparison of the HESPA 2015 Model (New) to the HEJA 2010 Model (Old)

Many of the HEJA Sub-competencies correlate to similar HESPA Sub-competencies. If the Sub-competency is worded the same in both Frameworks, it is <u>underlined</u>. All advanced-1 Sub-competencies are indicated by the symbol ❖, and the advanced-2 Sub-competencies are indicated by the symbol ■. "No Match" indicates no direct/similar Sub-competency.

KEY: entry level - no symbol; advanced 1 ❖; advanced 2 ■
Sub-competency worded the same in both Frameworks is <u>underlined</u>.

Area I: Assess Needs, Resources, and Capacity for Health Education/Promotion		
HESPA (New) Competencies and Sub-competencies		**Corresponding HEJA (Old) Competencies and Sub-competencies**
1.1	**Plan Assessment Process for Health Education/Promotion**	**1.1**
1.1.1	Define the priority population to be assessed	2.1.2, 6.2.3
1.1.2	Identify existing and necessary resources to conduct assessments	1.1.1
1.1.3	Engage priority populations, partners, and stakeholders to participate in the assessment process	1.1.2❖, 1.1.5❖
1.1.4❖	Apply theories and/or models to assessment process	1.1.3
1.1.5	Apply ethical principles to the assessment process	1.3.7
1.2	**Access Existing Information and Data Related to Health**	**1.2**
1.2.1	Identify sources of secondary data related to health	1.2.1, 1.2.6
1.2.2❖	Establish collaborative relationships and agreements that facilitate access to data	<u>1.2.5</u>
1.2.3	Review related literature	1.2.2
1.2.4	Identify gaps in the secondary data	1.2.4, 1.2.5
1.2.5	Extract data from existing databases	1.3.1
1.2.6	Determine the validity of existing data	1.2.3
1.3	**Collect Primary Data to Determine Needs**	**1.3**
1.3.1	Identify data collection instruments	1.3.3, 4.1.8
1.3.2	Select data collection methods for use in assessment	1.3.3, 1.3.4
1.3.3	Develop data collection procedures	1.1.4

Appendix B2: Comparison of the Competencies and Sub-competencies of the HESPA 2015 Model and the HEJA 2010 Model

KEY: entry level - no symbol; advanced 1 ❖; advanced 2 ■
Sub-competency worded the same in both Frameworks is <u>underlined</u>.

Area I: Assess Needs, Resources, and Capacity for Health Education/Promotion		
HESPA (New) Competencies and Sub-competencies		**Corresponding HEJA (Old) Competencies and Sub-competencies**
1.3.4	Train personnel assisting with data collection	1.3.5
1.3.5	Implement quantitative and/or qualitative data collection	1.3.6
1.4	**Analyze Relationships Among Behavioral, Environmental, and other Factors that Influence Health**	**1.4**
1.4.1	Identify and analyze factors that influence health behaviors	1.4.1, 1.4.2
1.4.2	Identify and analyze factors that impact health	1.4.3, 1.4.4
1.4.3	Identify the impact of emerging social, economic, and other trends on health	1.7.4
1.5	**Examine Factors that Influence the Process by Which People Learn**	**1.5**
1.5.1	Identify and analyze factors that foster or hinder the learning process	1.5.1, 1.5.2 ■
1.5.2	Identify and analyze factors that foster or hinder knowledge acquisition	1.5.1, 1.5.2 ■
1.5.3	Identify and analyze factors that influence attitudes and beliefs	1.5.3, 1.5.4
1.5.4	Identify and analyze factors that foster or hinder acquisition of skills	1.5.5, 1.5.6 ❖
1.6	**Examine Factors that Enhance or Impede the Process of Health Education/Promotion**	**1.6**
1.6.1	Determine the extent of available health education/promotion programs and interventions	1.6.1
1.6.2	Identify policies related to health education/promotion	1.6.1
1.6.3	Assess the effectiveness of existing health education/promotion programs and interventions	1.6.2
1.6.4	Assess social, environmental, political, and other factors that may impact health education/promotion	<u>1.6.4</u>
1.6.5	Analyze the capacity for providing necessary health education/promotion	<u>1.6.5</u>
1.7	**Determine Needs for Health Education/Promotion Based on Assessment Findings**	**1.7**
1.7.1 ❖	Synthesize assessment findings	1.7.2 ■
1.7.2	Identify current needs, resources, and capacity	1.6.6, 1.7.4
1.7.3	Prioritize health education/promotion needs	<u>1.7.3</u>

Appendix B2: Comparison of the Competencies and Sub-competencies of the HESPA 2015 Model and the HEJA 2010 Model

KEY: entry level - no symbol; advanced 1 ❖; advanced 2 ■
Sub-competency worded the same in both Frameworks is underlined.

Area I: Assess Needs, Resources, and Capacity for Health Education/Promotion		
HESPA (New) Competencies and Sub-competencies		**Corresponding HEJA (Old) Competencies and Sub-competencies**
1.7.4	Develop recommendations for health education/promotion based on assessment findings	2.1.1
1.7.5	Report assessment findings	<u>1.7.5</u>
Area II: Plan Health Education/Promotion		
2.1	**Involve Priority Populations, Partners, and other Stakeholders in the Planning Process**	<u>2.1</u>
2.1.1	Identify priority populations, partners, and other stakeholders	2.1.2, 6.2.3
2.1.2	Use strategies to convene priority populations, partners, and other stakeholders	2.1.1, 2.13
2.1.3	Facilitate collaborative efforts among priority populations, partners, and other stakeholders	2.1.4
2.1.4	Elicit input about the plan	2.1.5
2.1.5	Obtain commitments to participate in health education/promotion	2.1.6
2.2	**Develop Goals and Objectives**	<u>2.2</u>
2.2.1	Identify desired outcomes using the needs assessment results	2.2.1❖, <u>2.2.2</u>
2.2.2	Develop vision statement	New
2.2.3	Develop mission statement	5.2.6, 5.3.7
2.2.4	Develop goal statements	<u>2.2.4</u>
2.2.5	Develop specific, measurable, attainable, realistic, and time-sensitive objectives	2.2.5
2.3	**Select or Design Strategies/Interventions**	2.3
2.3.1❖	Select planning model(s) for health education/promotion	2.2.3 ■
2.3.2❖	Assess efficacy of various strategies/interventions to ensure consistency with objectives	2.3.1 ■
2.3.3❖	Apply principles of evidence-based practice in selecting and/or designing strategies/interventions	2.3.2, 2.3.3
2.3.4	Apply principles of cultural competence in selecting and/or designing strategies/interventions	<u>2.3.5</u>
2.3.5	Address diversity within priority populations in selecting and/or designing strategies/interventions	2.3.5

Appendix B2: Comparison of the Competencies and Sub-competencies of the HESPA 2015 Model and the HEJA 2010 Model

KEY: entry level - no symbol; advanced 1 ❖; advanced 2 ■
Sub-competency worded the same in both Frameworks is <u>underlined</u>.

Area II: Plan Health Education/Promotion		
HESPA (New) Competencies and Sub-competencies		**Corresponding HEJA (Old) Competencies and Sub-competencies**
2.3.6	Identify delivery methods and settings to facilitate learning	2.5.4
2.3.7	Tailor strategies/interventions for priority populations	7.2.2
2.3.8	Adapt existing strategies/interventions as needed	2.3.2, 6.2.6
2.3.9 ❖	Conduct pilot test of strategies/interventions	2.3.6
2.3.10 ❖	Refine strategies/interventions based on pilot feedback	2.5.3
2.3.11	Apply ethical principles in selecting strategies and designing interventions	2.3.4
2.3.12	Comply with legal standards in selecting strategies and designing interventions	2.3.4
2.4	**Develop a Plan for the Delivery of Health Education/Promotion**	**2.4**
2.4.1	Use theories and/or models to guide the delivery plan	2.4.3
2.4.2	Identify the resources involved in the delivery of health education/promotion	2.2.6, 2.4.2
2.4.3	Organize health education/promotion into a logical sequence	2.4.4 ❖
2.4.4	Develop a timeline for the delivery of health education/promotion	<u>2.4.5</u> ❖
2.4.5	Develop marketing plan to deliver health program	3.1.5
2.4.6	Select methods and/or channels for reaching priority populations	7.2.4
2.4.7	Analyze the opportunity for integrating health education/promotion into other programs	<u>2.4.6</u>
2.4.8 ❖	Develop a process for integrating health education/promotion into other programs when needed	2.4.7
2.4.9	Assess the sustainability of the delivery plan	7.3.3
2.4.10	Design and conduct pilot study of health education/promotion plan	2.3.6, 2.5.3
2.5	**Address Factors that Influence Implementation of Health Education/Promotion**	**2.5**
2.5.1	Identify and analyze factors that foster or hinder implementation	2.5.1, 2.5.2
2.5.2	Develop plans and processes to overcome potential barriers to implementation	2.5.3, 2.5.4

Appendix B2: Comparison of the Competencies and Sub-competencies of the HESPA 2015 Model and the HEJA 2010 Model

KEY: entry level - no symbol; advanced 1 ❖; advanced 2 ■
Sub-competency worded the same in both Frameworks is <u>underlined</u>.

Area III: Implement Health Education/Promotion		
HESPA (New) Competencies and Sub-competencies		**Corresponding HEJA (Old) Competencies and Sub-competencies**
3.1	**Coordinate Logistics Necessary to Implement Plan**	New
3.1.1	Create an environment conducive to learning	2.5.4
3.1.2	Develop materials to implement plan	New
3.1.3	Secure resources to implement plan	1.6.6, 2.4.2
3.1.4	Arrange for needed services to implement plan	New
3.1.5	Apply ethical principles to the implementation process	3.2.5
3.1.6	Comply with legal standards that apply to implementation	3.2.5
3.2	**Train Staff Members and Volunteers Involved in Implementation of Health Education/Promotion**	3.3
3.2.1❖	Develop training objectives	3.3.3❖
3.2.2	Recruit individuals needed for implementation	3.3.1
3.2.3❖	Identify training needs of individuals involved in implementation	3.3.2❖
3.2.4❖	Develop training using best practices	3.3.4❖, 3.3.5, 6.2.6❖
3.2.5❖	Implement training	3.3.6, 6.2.9
3.2.6❖	Provide support and technical assistance to those implementing the plan	New❖
3.2.7❖	Evaluate training	3.3.7❖, 6.2.10❖
3.2.8❖	Use evaluation findings to plan/modify future training	3.3.8❖
3.3	**Implement Health Education/Promotion Plan**	3.1
3.3.1	Collect baseline data	<u>3.1.2</u>
3.3.2❖	Apply theories and/or models of implementation	3.1.6
3.3.3	Assess readiness for implementation	<u>3.1.1</u>
3.3.4	Apply principles of diversity and cultural competence in implementing health education/promotion plan	3.1.3
3.3.5	Implement marketing plan	3.1.5
3.3.6	Deliver health education/promotion as designed	3.1.4, 3.1.7
3.3.7	Use a variety of strategies to deliver plan	<u>3.1.4</u>

Appendix B2: Comparison of the Competencies and Sub-competencies of the HESPA 2015 Model and the HEJA 2010 Model

KEY: entry level - no symbol; advanced 1 ❖; advanced 2 ■
Sub-competency worded the same in both Frameworks is <u>underlined</u>.

	Area III: Implement Health Education/Promotion	
	HESPA (New) Competencies and Sub-competencies	Corresponding HEJA (Old) Competencies and Sub-competencies
3.4	**Monitor Implementation of Health Education/Promotion**	3.2
3.4.1	Monitor progress in accordance with timeline progress in achieving objectives	<u>3.2.1</u>
3.4.2	Assess progress in achieving objectives	<u>3.2.2</u>
3.4.3	Ensure plan is implemented consistently	2.3.1
3.4.4	Modify plan when needed	3.2.3
3.4.5	Monitor use of resources	<u>3.2.4</u>
3.4.6	Evaluate sustainability of implementation	New
3.4.7	Ensure compliance with legal standards	3.2.5
3.4.8	Monitor adherence to ethical principles in the implementation of health education/promotion	3.2.5
	Area IV: Conduct Evaluation and Research Related to Health Education/Promotion	
4.1	**Develop Evaluation Plan for Health Education/Promotion**	4.1
4.1.1 ❖	Determine the purpose and goals of evaluation	4.1.1 ■
4.1.2 ❖	Develop questions to be answered by the evaluation	4.1.2 ■
4.1.3 ❖	Create a logic model to guide the evaluation process	4.1.11 ■
4.1.4 ❖	Adapt/modify a logic model to guide the evaluation process	4.1.11 ■
4.1.5 ❖	Assess needed and available resources to conduct evaluation	4.1.3
4.1.6 ❖	Determine the types of data (for example, qualitative, quantitative) to be collected	4.1.6, 4.1.7 ■
4.1.7 ❖	Select a model for evaluation	New
4.1.8 ❖	Develop data collection procedures for evaluation	1.3.4
4.1.9 ■	Develop data analysis plan for evaluation	<u>4.1.12</u>
4.1.10 ❖	Apply ethical principles to the evaluation process	4.1.14, 4.3.5
4.2	**Develop a Research Plan for Health Education/Promotion**	4.1
4.2.1 ■	Create statement of purpose	4.1.1
4.2.2 ■	Assess feasibility of conducting research	4.1.3
4.2.3 ■	Conduct search for related literature	1.2.6, 4.1.4, 4.1.5

Appendix B2: Comparison of the Competencies and Sub-competencies of the HESPA 2015 Model and the HEJA 2010 Model

KEY: entry level - no symbol; advanced 1 ❖; advanced 2 ■
Sub-competency worded the same in both Frameworks is <u>underlined</u>.

Area IV: Conduct Evaluation and Research Related to Health Education/Promotion		
HESPA (New) Competencies and Sub-competencies		Corresponding HEJA (Old) Competencies and Sub-competencies
4.2.4 ■	Analyze and synthesize information found in the literature	4.1.4, 4.1.5
4.2.5 ■	Develop research questions and/or hypotheses	4.1.2 ■
4.2.6 ■	Assess the merits and limitations of qualitative and quantitative data collection	4.1.6, 4.1.7 ■
4.2.7 ■	Select research design to address the research questions	New
4.2.8 ■	Determine suitability of existing data collection instruments	1.3.3, 4.1.8
4.2.9 ■	Identify research participants	New
4.2.10 ■	Develop sampling plan to select participants	New
4.2.11 ■	Develop data collection procedures for research	New
4.2.12 ■	Develop data analysis plan for research	4.1.13 ■
4.2.13 ■	Develop a plan for non-respondent follow-up	New
4.2.14 ■	Apply ethical principles to the research process	4.1.14
4.3 ■	**Select, Adapt and/or Create Instruments to Collect Data**	**4.2**
4.3.1 ■	Identify existing data collection instruments	1.3.3, <u>4.1.8</u>, 4.1.9 4.1.10 ■
4.3.2 ■	Adapt/modify existing data collection instruments	1.3.4, 4.19, 4.1.10 ■
4.3.3 ■	Create new data collection instruments	1.3.4
4.3.4	Identify useable items from existing instruments	1.3.4, 4.2.1
4.3.5	Adapt/modify existing items	1.3.4, 4.2.2, 4.2.3 ■
4.3.6 ■	Create new items to be used in data collection	1.3.4, 4.2.2, 4.2.3 ■
4.3.7 ■	Pilot test data collection instrument	1.3.4
4.3.8 ■	Establish validity of data collection instruments	1.3.4, <u>4.2.4</u>
4.3.9 ■	Ensure that data collection instruments generate reliable data	1.3.4, 4.2.5
4.3.10 ■	Ensure fairness of data collection instruments (for example, reduce bias, use language appropriate to priority population)	New

Appendix B2: Comparison of the Competencies and Sub-competencies of the HESPA 2015 Model and the HEJA 2010 Model

KEY: entry level - no symbol; advanced 1 ❖; advanced 2 ■
Sub-competency worded the same in both Frameworks is underlined.

Area IV: Conduct Evaluation and Research Related to Health Education/Promotion		
HESPA (New) Competencies and Sub-competencies		**Corresponding HEJA (Old) Competencies and Sub-competencies**
4.4	**Collect and Manage Data**	**4.3**
4.4.1 ■	Train data collectors involved in evaluation and/or research	4.3.1
4.4.2 ■	Collect data based on the evaluation or research plan	4.3.1
4.4.3	Monitor and manage data collection	4.3.2
4.4.4	Use available technology to collect, monitor and manage data	4.3.2
4.4.5	Comply with laws and regulations when collecting, storing, and protecting participant data	4.3.5, 5.3.5
4.5	**Analyze Data**	**4.3**
4.5.1 ■	Prepare data for analysis	New
4.5.2 ❖	Analyze data using qualitative methods	4.3.4
4.5.3 ■	Analyze data using descriptive statistical methods	4.3.3
4.5.4 ■	Analyze data using inferential statistical methods	4.3.3
4.5.5 ■	Use technology to analyze data	New
4.6	**Interpret Results**	**4.4**
4.6.1 ■	Synthesize the analyzed data	5.2.4 ■
4.6.2 ■	Explain how the results address the questions and/or hypotheses	4.3.3, 4.4.1
4.6.3 ■	Compare findings to results from other studies or evaluations	4.4.2
4.6.4 ■	Propose possible explanations of findings	<u>4.4.3</u>
4.6.5 ■	Identify limitations of findings	4.4.4
4.6.6 ■	Address delimitations as they relate to findings	4.4.4
4.6.7 ■	Draw conclusions based on findings	4.4.3
4.6.8 ■	Develop recommendations based on findings	4.4.5
4.7	**Apply Findings**	**4.5**
4.7.1	Communicate findings to priority populations, partners, and stakeholders	4.5.1
4.7.2	Solicit feedback from priority populations, partners, and stakeholders	4.5.1

Appendix B2: Comparison of the Competencies and Sub-competencies of the HESPA 2015 Model and the HEJA 2010 Model

KEY: entry level - no symbol; advanced 1 ❖; advanced 2 ■
Sub-competency worded the same in both Frameworks is <u>underlined</u>.

Area IV: Conduct Evaluation and Research Related to Health Education/Promotion		
HESPA (New) Competencies and Sub-competencies		**Corresponding HEJA (Old) Competencies and Sub-competencies**
4.7.33	Evaluate feasibility of implementing recommendations	4.5.2 ■
4.7.4	Incorporate findings into program improvement and refinement	4.5.3
4.7.5 ■	Disseminate findings using a variety of methods	4.5.4 ■
Area V: Administer and Manage Health Education/Promotion		
5.1	**Manage Financial Resources for Health Education/Promotion Programs**	**5.1**
5.1.1 ❖	Develop financial plan	New
5.1.2 ❖	Evaluate financial needs and resources	7.1.2
5.1.3 ❖	Identify internal and/or external funding sources	5.1.1 ❖
5.1.4 ❖	Prepare budget requests	5.1.2 ❖
5.1.5 ❖	Develop program budgets	5.1.3 ❖
5.1.6 ❖	Manage program budgets	<u>5.1.4 ❖</u>
5.1.7 ❖	Conduct cost analysis for programs	New
5.1.8 ❖	Prepare budget reports	<u>5.1.5 ❖</u>
5.1.9 ❖	Monitor financial plan	New
5.1.10 ❖	Create requests for funding proposals	New
5.1.11 ❖	Write grant proposals	New
5.1.12	Conduct reviews of funding proposals	New
5.1.13 ❖	Apply ethical principles when managing financial resources	5.1.6 ❖
5.2	**Manage Technology Resources**	**New**
5.2.1	Assess technology needs to support health education/promotion	7.3.2
5.2.2	Use technology to collect, store and retrieve program management data	5.2.4 ❖
5.2.3	Apply ethical principles in managing technology resources	New
5.2.4	Evaluate emerging technologies for applicability to health education/promotion	7.1.1, 7.4.7

Appendix B2: Comparison of the Competencies and Sub-competencies of the HESPA 2015 Model and the HEJA 2010 Model

KEY: entry level - no symbol; advanced 1 ❖; advanced 2 ■
Sub-competency worded the same in both Frameworks is underlined.

Area V: Administer and Manage Health Education/Promotion		
HESPA (New) Competencies and Sub-competencies		Corresponding HEJA (Old) Competencies and Sub-competencies
5.3	**Manage Relationships with Partners and other Stakeholders**	5.5
5.3.1	Assess capacity of partners and other stakeholders to meet program goals	5.5.1 ❖, 5.5.2 ❖
5.3.2 ❖	Facilitate discussions with partners and other stakeholders regarding program resource needs	5.2.2 ❖, 5.3.3 ❖, 5.5.3
5.3.3	Create agreements (for example, memoranda of understanding) with partners and other stakeholders	1.2.5, 5.2.2 ❖, 5.3.3 ❖, 5.5.3, 6.3.6
5.3.4	Monitor relationships with partners and other stakeholders	5.5.3, 5.5.4
5.3.5 ❖	Elicit feedback from partners and other stakeholders	5.5.4 ❖
5.3.6 ❖	Evaluate relationships with partners and other stakeholders	5.5.5 ❖
5.4	**Gain Acceptance and Support for Health Education/Promotion Programs**	5.2
5.4.1	Demonstrate how programs align with organizational structure, mission, and goals	5.2.3 ❖, 5.2.6
5.4.2	Identify evidence to justify programs	5.2.3 ❖
5.4.3	Create a rationale to gain or maintain program support	5.2.1 ❖, 5.2.3 ❖
5.4.4	Use various communication strategies to present rationale	5.2.1 ❖, 5.2.3 ❖
5.5	**Demonstrate Leadership**	5.3
5.5.1 ❖	Facilitate efforts to achieve organizational mission	5.3.7
5.5.2	Analyze an organization's culture to determine the extent to which it supports health education/promotion	5.3.2
5.5.3	Develop strategies to reinforce or change organizational culture to support health education/promotion	5.3.4
5.5.4 ❖	Facilitate needed changes to organizational culture	5.3.9
5.5.5 ❖	Conduct strategic planning	5.3.1
5.5.6 ❖	Implement strategic plan	5.3.1
5.5.7 ❖	Monitor strategic plan	5.3.1
5.5.8	Conduct program quality assurance/process improvement	5.3.8
5.5.9	Comply with existing laws and regulations	5.3.5
5.5.10	Adhere to ethical principles of the profession	5.3.6

Appendix B2: Comparison of the Competencies and Sub-competencies of the HESPA 2015 Model and the HEJA 2010 Model

KEY: entry level - no symbol; advanced 1 ❖; advanced 2 ■
Sub-competency worded the same in both Frameworks is <u>underlined</u>.

Area V: Administer and Manage Health Education/Promotion		
HESPA (New) Competencies and Sub-competencies		Corresponding HEJA (Old) Competencies and Sub-competencies
5.6	Manage Human Resources for Health Education/Promotion Programs	5.4
5.6.1 ❖	Assess staffing needs	New
5.6.2 ❖	Develop job descriptions	5.4.1
5.6.3 ❖	Apply human resource policies consistent with laws and regulations	5.4.2., 5.4.3, 5.4.4
5.6.4 ❖	Evaluate qualifications of staff members and volunteers needed for programs	5.4.4
5.6.5	Recruit staff members and volunteers for programs	5.4.5
5.6.6 ❖	Determine staff member and volunteer professional development needs	New
5.6.7 ❖	Develop strategies to enhance staff member and volunteer professional development	5.4.9 ❖
5.6.8 ❖	Implement strategies to enhance the professional development of staff members and volunteers	5.2.5, 5.4.10 ❖
5.6.9 ❖	Develop and implement strategies to retain staff members and volunteers	New
5.6.10 ❖	Employ conflict resolution techniques	5.4.6
5.6.11 ❖	Facilitate team development	5.4.7
5.6.12 ❖	Evaluate performance of staff members and volunteers	5.4.11
5.6.13 ❖	Monitor performance and/or compliance of funding recipients	New
5.6.14 ❖	Apply ethical principles when managing human resources	5.4.2, 5.4.8
Area VI: Serve as a Health Education/Promotion Resource Person		
6.1	**Obtain and Disseminate Health-Related Information**	**6.1**
6.1.1	Assess needs for health-related information	6.1.1
6.1.2	Identify valid information resources	1.2.3, 6.1.2, 6.1.3
6.1.3	Evaluate resource materials for accuracy, relevance, and timeliness	6.1.3
6.1.4	Adapt information for consumer	6.1.4, 6.1.5
6.1.5	Convey health-related information to consumer	6.1.4, 6.1.5

Appendix B2: Comparison of the Competencies and Sub-competencies of the HESPA 2015 Model and the HEJA 2010 Model

KEY: entry level - no symbol; advanced 1 ❖; advanced 2 ■
Sub-competency worded the same in both Frameworks is <u>underlined</u>.

Area VI: Serve as a Health Education/Promotion Resource Person		
HESPA (New) Competencies and Sub-competencies		**Corresponding HEJA (Old) Competencies and Sub-competencies**
6.2	**Train Others to Use Health Education/Promotion Skills**	6.2
6.2.1 ❖	Assess training needs of potential participants	6.2.1 ❖, 6.2.4 ❖,
6.2.2 ❖	Develop a plan for conducting training	6.2.2 ❖, 6.2.7 ❖
6.2.3 ❖	Identify resources needed to conduct training	6.2.5 ❖
6.2.4 ❖	Implement planned training	6.2.8 ❖, 6.2.9 ❖
6.2.5 ❖	Conduct formative and summative evaluations of training	6.2.9 ❖, 6.2.10 ❖
6.2.6 ❖	Use evaluative feedback to create future trainings	
6.3	**Provide Advice and Consultation on Health Education/Promotion Issues**	6.3
6.3.1 ❖	Assess and prioritize requests for advice/consultation	6.3.1, 6.3.2
6.3.2 ❖	Establish advisory/consultative relationships	6.3.3, 6.3.4
6.3.3 ❖	Provide expert assistance and guidance	6.3.5 ❖
6.3.4 ❖	Evaluate the effectiveness of the expert assistance provided	<u>6.3.7 ❖</u>
6.3.5 ❖	Apply ethical principles in consultative relationships	<u>6.3.8</u>
Area VII: Communicate, Promote, and Advocate for Health, Health Education/Promotion, and the Profession		
7.1	**Identify, Develop, and Deliver Messages Using a Variety of Communication Strategies, Methods, and Techniques**	7.2, 7.3
7.1.1	Create messages using communication theories and/or models	<u>7.2.1</u>
7.1.2	Identify level of literacy of intended audience	New
7.1.3	Tailor messages for intended audience	7.2.2
7.1.4 ❖	Pilot test messages and delivery methods	7.2.5
7.1.5 ❖	Revise messages based on pilot feedback	<u>7.2.6</u>
7.1.6	Assess and select methods and technologies used to deliver messages	7.2.4
7.1.7	Deliver messages using media and communication strategies	7.2.3, 7.2.4, 7.3.1
7.1.8	Evaluate the impact of the delivered messages	New

Appendix B2: Comparison of the Competencies and Sub-competencies of the HESPA 2015 Model and the HEJA 2010 Model

KEY: entry level - no symbol; advanced 1 ❖; advanced 2 ■
Sub-competency worded the same in both Frameworks is <u>underlined</u>.

Area VII: Communicate, Promote, and Advocate for Health, Health Education/Promotion, and the Profession		
HESPA (New) Competencies and Sub-competencies		**Corresponding HEJA (Old) Competencies and Sub-competencies**
7.2	**Engage in Advocacy for Health and Health Education/Promotion**	**7.4**
7.2.1	Identify current and emerging issues requiring advocacy	7.1.1
7.2.2	Engage stakeholders in advocacy initiatives	7.4.1
7.2.3	Access resources (for example, financial, personnel, information, data) related to identified advocacy needs	7.4.1, 7.4.5
7.2.4	Develop advocacy plans in compliance with local, state, and/or federal policies and procedures	<u>7.4.2</u>
7.2.5	Use strategies that advance advocacy goals	7.4.5, 7.4.7, 7.5.1 ■, 7.5.3
7.2.6	Implement advocacy plans	<u>7.4.6</u>
7.2.7	Evaluate advocacy efforts	7.4.10 ■
7.2.8	Comply with organizational policies related to participating in advocacy	<u>7.4.3</u>
7.2.9	Lead advocacy initiatives related to health	7.4.4, 7.4.8, 7.4.9 ■
7.3	**Influence Policy and/or Systems Change to Promote Health and Health Education**	**7.5**
7.3.1	Assess the impact of existing and proposed policies on health	7.1.3, 7.5.1 ■
7.3.2	Assess the impact of existing and proposed policies on health education	7.5.1
7.3.3	Assess the impact of existing systems on health	5.3.8
7.3.4	Project the impact of proposed systems changes on health education	5.3.8
7.3.5	Use evidence-based findings in policy analysis	7.5.1 ■, 7.5.4 ■
7.3.6 ❖	Develop policies to promote health using evidence-based findings	7.5.4 ■
7.3.7 ❖	Identify factors that influence decision-makers	7.1.4
7.3.8 ❖	Use policy advocacy techniques to influence decision-makers	7.1.4, 7.5.5
7.3.9	Use media advocacy techniques to influence decision-makers	7.1.14, 7.5.5
7.3.10	Engage in legislative advocacy	7.4.8, 7.5.3

Appendix B2: Comparison of the Competencies and Sub-competencies of the HESPA 2015 Model and the HEJA 2010 Model

KEY: entry level - no symbol; advanced 1 ❖; advanced 2 ■
Sub-competency worded the same in both Frameworks is <u>underlined</u>.

Area VII: Communicate, Promote, and Advocate for Health, Health Education/Promotion, and the Profession		
HESPA (New) Competencies and Sub-competencies		**Corresponding HEJA (Old) Competencies and Sub-competencies**
7.4	**Promote the Health Education Profession**	**7.6**
7.4.1	Explain the major responsibilities of the health education specialist	7.6.2, 7.6.3
7.4.2	Explain the role of professional organizations in advancing the profession	<u>7.6.4</u>
7.4.3	Explain the benefits of participating in professional organizations	<u>7.6.5</u>
7.4.4	Advocate for professional development of health education specialists	7.6.6
7.4.5	Advocate for the profession	7.6.5
7.4.6	Explain the history of the profession and its current and future implications for professional practice	7.6.7
7.4.7	Explain the role of credentialing (for example, individual, program) in the promotion of the profession	7.6.8
7.4.8	Develop and implement a professional development plan	7.6.1, 7.6.9
7.4.9 ■	Serve as a mentor to others in the profession	7.6.10
7.4.10 ■	Develop materials that contribute to the professional literature	7.6.11
7.4.11 ■	Engage in service to advance the profession	7.6.12

Appendix C: History of Working Groups for Health Education Specialist Competency Development

Committees, task forces, and other working groups who contributed to the HESPA 2015 are listed here. Various committees of HESPA 2015, HEJA 2010, CUP, and previous committees who worked on defining the role and Competencies of health education specialists are also listed.

Health Education Specialist Practice Analysis [HESPA] 2015 (2013-2014)

Professional Examination Service
Carla M. Caro, MA
Patricia M. Muenzen, MA
Dianne Henderson-Montero, PhD

NCHEC Support Staff
Cynthia S. Kusorgbor-Narh, MPH, CHES

HESPA 2015 Steering Committee
M. Elaine Auld, MPH, MCHES
Dixie Dennis, PhD, MCHES
Eva I. Doyle, PhD, MSEd, MCHES
Linda Lysoby, MS, MCHES, CAE
James F. McKenzie, PhD, MPH, MCHES

HESPA 2015 Task Force
Dixie Dennis, PhD, MCHES (Co-chair)
James F. McKenzie, PhD, MPH, MCHES (Co-chair)
Kelly Brennan, MEd, MCHES
Annie L. Dickerson, MA, CHES
Michele Guadalupe, MPH
Gilberto Hernandez, MA, CHES
Michael Staufacker, MA, MCHES
Grace Salako Smith, PhD, CHES
Alyson Taub, PhD, MCHES
Linh Tran, BS, CHES
Starr Wharton, MS, MCHES
Alexis Williams, MPH, CHES

HESPA 2015 Telephone Interview Panel
David Birch, PhD, MCHES
Karen Cottrell, MEd
Gary D. Gilmore, PhD, MPH, MCHES
Susan Goekler, PhD, MCHES;
Madonna Lynn Holbrook-Lowe, MPH, MCHES
Garry M. Lindsay, MPH, MCHES
Michael McNeil, MS, EdD, CHES
Sarah J. Olson, MS, CHES
Dan Perales, DrPH, MPH
Susan M. Radius, PhD, MCHES
Robert F. Valois MS, PhD, MPH, FAAHB

HESPA 2015 Independent Review Panel
Christine Abarca, MPH, MCHES
Leititia Bailey, MPH, CHES
Srijana M. Bajrachrya, PhD, MCHES
Mario C Browne, MPH, CHES
Brenda Carter
Blanche Collins, MHSE, MCHES
Sonja Davis, BS, CHES
Bonnie J. Edmondson, Ed.D, MS
Richard Edwards, PhD, CHES
Jim Grizzell, MA, MBA, MCHES
Stacy Haitsuka, MPH, CHES
Maureen W. Krouse, BS, CHES
Teresa Lovely, MS, MCHES
Carol Noel Michaels, MPH, MCHES
Chanita W. Neal, MHSE, CHES
Larry Olsen, DrPH, MCHES
Patricia G. Owen, MCHES
Tamara Oyola-Santiago, MPH, CHES
Carrie Shult, MHS, CHES
Robert Walker, PhD, MS

Appendix C: History of Working Groups for Health Education Specialist Competency Development

HESPA 2015 Pilot Test Participants
David Brown, EdD MCHES
Yyolany Caffrey, MPH, CHES
Lisa Clough, MSEd, CHES
Emily Dunnebacke, BS, CHES
Jody Early, PhD, MCHES
Amanda Graves, BSEd, MCHES
Jake Hanson, BS, CHES
Patty Holman, MS, CHES
Katie Jourdan, MPH, CHES
Sarojini Kanotra, PhD, CHES
Emily Lee, MEd, CHES
Lindsey Mitchell, MPH
Charlotte Petonic, BS, CHES
Janet Pryor, BS
Estelle Raboni, MPH, MCHES
Krista Reale, MA, CHES
Patti Rittling, PhD, CHES
Keiko Sakagami, EdD, MCHES
Kimberley Sinclair, MPH
Caile Spear, PhD, MCHES
Chelsea Stone, BS, CHES
Jerah Thomas, MPH, CHES
Chantay Williams, MPH
Holly Wilson, MHSE, CHES

National Health Educator Job Analysis [HEJA] 2010 (2008-2009) Professional Examination Service
Carla M. Caro, MA
Patricia M. Muenzen, MA

HEJA 2010 Steering Committee
M. Elaine Auld, MPH, CHES
Eva I. Doyle, PhD, MSEd, CHES
Linda Lysoby, MS, CHES, CAE
Beverly Saxton Mahoney, RN, MS, PhD, CHES
Becky J. Smith, PhD, CHES, CAE

HEJA 2010 Task Force
Eva I. Doyle, PhD, MSEd, CHES (Chair)
Kelly Bishop Alley, MA, CHES
Chesley Cheatham, MEd, CHES
Lillie M. Hall, MPH, CHES
Mary Marks, PhD
James F. McKenzie, PhD, MPH, CHES
Michael P. McNeil, MS, CHES
Darcy Scharff, PhD
Michael Staufacker, MA, CHES
Alyson Taub, PhD, CHES
Carol A. Younkin, RN, MA, CHES

HEJA 2010 Telephone Interview Panel
John Allegrante, PhD
Nancy Atmospera-Walch, RN, BSN, MPH, CHES
Karen Cottrell, MEd
Gary Gilmore, PhD, MPH, CHES
James Grizzell, MA, MBA, CHES
Pamela Hoalt, PhD, LPC
Jacqueline Valenzuela, MPH, CHES
Louise Villejo, MPH, CHES
C. Lynn Woodhouse, EdD, MPH

HEJA 2010 Independent Review Panel
Edith Cabuslay, MPH
Elizabeth H. Chaney, PhD, CHES
Dixie L. Dennis, PhD, CHES
Marcy Harrington, MPA, CHES
Jon W. Hisgen, MS, CHES
Judith A. Johns, MS, CHES
Linda LaSalle, PhD
Garry M. Lindsay, MPH, CHES
Kimberley McBride, MPH
Larry K. Olsen, DrPH, CHES
Deyonne M. Sandoval, MS, CHES
Audrey E. Shively, MSHSE, CHES
Rob Simmons, DrPH, MPH, CHES
Cortney E. Smith, MS, CHES
Virginia Smyly, MPH, CHES
Francisco Soto Mas, MD, PhD, MPH
Jody R. Steinhardt, MPH, CHES

Appendix C: History of Working Groups for Health Education Specialist Competency Development

HEJA 2010 Pilot Test Participants
Dori Babcock, MA
Janet Baggett, MA, CHES
Christine E. Beyer, PhD
Johanna Chase, MA, CHES
Chia-Ching Chen, EdD, CHES
Lori Elmore, MPH, CHES
Brian F. Geiger, PhD
Amanda Greene, PhD, CHES
Harpreet Grewal, MPH, CHES
Brent Hartman, MPH, CHES
Marissa Howat, CHES
Bernie Jarriel, MA, CHES
Raffy R. Luquis, PhD, CHES
Grace Miranda, MA, CHES
Brandy Peterson, MPH, CHES
Tywanna Purkett, MA, CHES
Susie Robinson, PhD, CHES
Keiko Sakagami, EdD, CHES
Jennifer Scofield, MA, CHES
Jody Vogelzang, PhD, CHES
Cathy D. Whaley, MA, CHES

Authors and Editors of *A Competency-Based Framework for Health Education Specialists – 2010*
Chris Arthur, PhD, CHES
Donna Beal, MPH, CHES
Cam Escoffery, PhD, MPH, CHES
Patricia A. Frye, DrPH, MPA, CHES;
Melissa Grim, PhD, CHES (author/editor)
Leonard Jack, Jr., PhD, MSc, CHES (author/editor)
Dennis Kamholtz, PhD, CHES
Maurice "Bud" Martin, PhD, CHES
Beverly Saxton Mahoney, RN, MS, PhD, CHES
James F. McKenzie, PhD, MPH, CHES
Angela Mickalide, PhD, CHES
Jacquie Rainey, DrPH, CHES
Rebecca Reeve, PhD, CHES
Christopher N. Thomas, MS, CHES
Tung-Sung "Sam" Tseng, DrPH, MS, CHES
Kelly Wilson, PhD, CHES
Katherine Wilson, PhD, CHES

National Health Educator Competencies Update Project [CUP] (1998-2004)

CUP Steering Committee
Dr. Gary Gilmore, CUP Chair
Dr. Larry Olsen
Dr. Alyson Taub

CUP Advisory Committee
Ms. Elaine Auld
Dr. David R. Black
Dr. Tom Butler
Dr. Ellen M. Capwell
Dr. Helen Welle Graf
Ms. Barbara Hager
Ms. Linda Lysoby
Dr. Beverly Mahoney
Dr. Mary Marks
Dr. Marion Micke
Dr. Kathleen Miner
Dr. Sheila M. Patterson
Dr. Susan Radius
Dr. Edmund Ricci
Dr. John Sciacca
Dr. Becky Smith
Dr. Margaret Smith
Dr. Carol Soha
Ms. Lori Stegmier
Dr. Stephen H. Stewart
Ms. Emily Tyler

CUP Data Analysis Group
Dr. Randy Black
Dr. Dave Connell
Dr. Dan Coster
Dr. Gary Gilmore
Dr. Kathy Miner
Dr. Larry Olsen
Dr. Alyson Taub

Appendix C: History of Working Groups for Health Education Specialist Competency Development

Graduate-Level Preparation Standards Project (1992-1998)

Joint Committee for the Development of Graduate-Level Preparation Standards
Dr. Margaret M. Smith and
Dr. Stephen H. Stewart, Co-Chairpersons
Dr. Evelyn E. Ames
Dr. Donald L. Calitri
Dr. William B. Cissell
Ms. Patricia P. Evans
Ms. Mary E. Hawkins
Mr. Douglas Rippler
Dr. Mark J. Kittleson
Dr. William C. Livingood, Jr.
Capt. Patricia D. Mail
Dr. Carl J. Peter
Dr. Donald A. Read
Ms. Ruth Richards
Dr. James Robinson III
Dr. Elaine M. Vitello

Graduate Competencies Writing Ad Hoc Committee
Ms. Patricia P. Evans
Dr. William C. Livingood, Jr.
Capt. Patricia D. Mail
Dr. James Robinson
Dr. Margaret M. Smith
Dr. Alyson Taub

Graduate Competencies Implementation Committee
Ms. Elaine Auld
Dr. Ellen M. Capwell
Dr. William B. Cissell
Mr. William B. Cosgrove
Ms. Patricia P. Evans
Ms. Aileen Frazee
Dr. Gary D. Gilmore
Dr. Audrey Gotsch
Dr. William C. Livingood, Jr.
Dr. Sheila M. Patterson
Dr. James Robinson
Dr. Louis Rowitz
Dr. Becky J. Smith
Dr. Margaret M. Smith
Dr. Stephen H. Stewart
Dr. Alyson Taub
Dr. Elaine M. Vitello

National Task Force on the Preparation and Practice of Health Educators (1978-1988)

Chair and Founder
Dr. Helen Cleary

Vice Chair and Co-founder
Dr. Peter Cortese

Original Task Force Members
Dr. Helen Cleary
Dr. Peter Cortese
Dr. John Burt
Dr. William Carlyon
Dr. Mabel Robinson
Dr. Helen S. Ross
Dr. Warren Schaller
Dr. Joan M. Wolle

Task Force Members
Dr. William B. Cissell
Dr. John Cooper
Dr. Bryan Cooke
Dr. Robert H. Conn
Dr. Wanda H. Judd
Ms. Elizabeth Lee
Rev. Robert McEwen
Ms. Helen Savage
Dr. Becky J. Smith
Mr. Leonard Tritsch
Dr. Alyson Taub
Dr. Elaine M. Vitello
Ms. Anna Skiff, MPH, Volunteer Staff

Appendix D: Competency Matrices

This section contains matrices that can be used by faculty members in university programs to evaluate the degree to which their curricula address the Areas of Responsibility, Competencies, and Sub-competencies of the HESPA 2015 Model. The faculty members can use the completed matrices to identify specific courses in which the Model components are addressed and the extent to which each Competency and Sub-competency is addressed within courses and across the curriculum. Identified gaps in coverage can be targeted for improvement. The results can be included in accreditation reports and communicated to students in the program who are interested in understanding program strengths and learning expectations.

Directions for Use of the Area of Responsibility Matrices

A matrix is provided in this section for each of the Seven Areas of Responsibility. Each Area of Responsibility matrix contains grids specific to the entry- and advanced-level Sub-competencies for that Area. Specific recommendations to the profession that impact curricula development can be found in Section IV of this publication. Baccalaureate degree programs should prepare graduates to perform all entry-level Competencies and Sub-competencies within the Areas of Responsibility. Master's and doctoral degree programs should prepare graduates to perform all entry- and advanced-level Competencies and Sub-competencies within the Areas of Responsibility. Additionally, doctoral programs should place additional emphasis on all advanced 2-level Sub-competencies. Due to the hierarchical nature of the HESPA 2015 Model (advanced-level building on entry-level), when evaluating a program designed to prepare students for advanced-level practice, some courses will need to be listed in the entry-level grid on the matrix to indicate courses in which entry-level Sub-competencies are highlighted. Other courses will need to be listed in the advanced-level grid to indicate courses in which advanced-level Sub-competencies are emphasized. It is possible that some courses may need to be listed on both grids and that some advanced-level Sub-competencies may be addressed in a baccalaureate degree program.

To use the matrices effectively, enter the course number and title of each professional preparation course required of health education majors enrolled in your program. Only faculty members currently responsible for teaching a course should rate a course. The designated course instructor(s) for a course should refer to the Competencies and Sub-competencies specific to each Area of Responsibility and determine whether or not each of the Sub-competencies is currently being taught as an integral part of the course. In making this determination, the course instructor(s) should note that a Competency statement does not merely represent subject matter relevant to a skill. The statement must be viewed as an actual Competency (i.e., skills and abilities). The question each instructor must answer in connection with every Competency and Sub-competency specified in the Area matrices is: "Are the students taking this course merely learning associated subject matter or are they learning to perform the described Competency (i.e., skills and abilities)?" Obviously, the instructor of each course is more qualified than any other faculty member to make that judgment.

If a Sub-competency is given major emphasis as part of a course, the instructor should place the number 2 in the corresponding box. If the Sub-competency receives at least minor study and practice in the course, the number 1 should be assigned. In the event that a Sub-competency is not a part of the content of that course, a score of 0 should be assigned. The total mathematical sum of these entries for each course should be recorded in the far right column titled "Total by Course." Figure D.1 contains example entries for four health education courses.

Appendix D: Competency Matrices

Area of Responsibility I Matrix
Area I: Assess Needs, Resources, and Capacity for Health Education/Promotion

Course Title	Comp 1.1 Sub-comp					Comp 1.2 Sub-comp						Comp 1.3 Sub-comp					Comp 1.4 Sub-comp			Comp 1.5 Sub-comp				Comp 1.6 Sub-comp					Comp 1.7 Sub-comp					Total by Course (Max=60)*
	.1	.2	.3	.4	.5	.1	.2	.3	.4	.5	.6	.1	.2	.3	.4	.5	.1	.2	.3	.1	.2	.3	.4	.1	.2	.3	.4	.5	.1	.2	.3	.4	.5	
Community Health	1	1	2	2	2	1	1	1	0	0	0	1	1	1	0	1	1	1	1	2	2	2	2	2	1	2	2	2	2	2	2	1	1	37
Biostatistics	1	0	1	1	1	1	0	1	1	2	2	1	1	0	1	1	2	2	1	2	1	1	0	0	0	0	0	0	0	0	0	0	1	21
Administration of H.E.	0	0	0	0	1	1	1	1	1	2	0	0	0	0	2	0	1	1	1	2	2	2	2	2	2	2	2	2	2	2	2	2	2	36
School Health	1	1	1	1	1	1	1	1	0	0	0	1	1	0	1	0	1	1	0	2	2	2	2	2	1	2	1	1	2	2	2	1	1	31

Total by Area of Responsibility*
Should not exceed maximum (60) x number of courses

Advanced 1-level

Course Title	Comp 1.1 Sub-comp .4	Comp 1.2 Sub-comp .2	Comp 1.7 Sub-comp .1	Total by Course (Max = 6)

Total by Area of Responsibility
Should not exceed maximum (6) x number of courses

Codes: 2=Major Emphasis, 1=Minor Emphasis, 0=No Emphasis; *Max: Maximum number possible per course
^No advanced 2-level Sub-competencies exist for Area of Responsibility I

Figure D.1 Example of Area of Responsibility Matrix Analysis

Appendix D: Competency Matrices

Directions for Use of the Analysis Sheets

When all of the Area of Responsibility matrices have been completed, the analysis sheets for entry-, advanced 1-, and advanced 2-levels should be used as an organizing and summarizing tool (see end of Appendix D). The analysis sheets are designed to facilitate organization of the combined data obtained by means of the Area of Responsibility matrices. The same courses that appeared on the Area of Responsibility matrices are listed along the vertical axis. The data recorded on the matrices should be transferred to the analysis sheets and used to identify strengths and potential areas for improvement in the curriculum.

Notice that for each Area of Responsibility, the Competencies are indicated by a numbering system with the first number indicating the Area of Responsibility and the second number indicating the specific Competency within that area (for example, Competency 1.1, Competency 1.2, Competency 1.3) across the horizontal axis. Below each Competency number is the total number of supportive Sub-competencies for that Competency. (In the entry-level analysis sheet, see Sub-competencies 4, 5, 5, 3, 4, 5, and 4 for Area of Responsibility I.)

In each completed Area of Responsibility matrix and for every course listed, enter the number of Sub-competencies given a rating of 2 and the number of those given a rating of 1 in the appropriate box (see Figure D.2). As an example, note in Figure D.1 that of four Sub-competencies specified as essential to the achievement of Competency 1.1 at the entry-level, the instructor of the community health course has reported that two Sub-competencies receive major emphasis (2), a third Sub-competency is given at least some emphasis (1), and the fourth Sub-competency is given no emphasis (0). In the analysis sheet (Figure D.2), the number of Sub-competencies given major emphasis (in this case, 2) is entered in the top portion of the box, and the number given minor emphasis (which is 1) is entered in the lower portion, so that it looks like a fraction (2/1).

As another example, for Competency 1.1, which contains four entry-level Sub-competencies, none is reported in Figure D.1 as being given major or minor emphasis in the Administration of Health Education (H.E.) course. For this reason, a 0 (zero) is entered for each Sub-competency in Figure D.1. Because there are neither 2s nor 1s reported in Figure D.1, the "fraction" in Figure D.2 is 0/0.

When all of the data have been entered into the analysis sheet (Figure D.2) for all of the courses, total and enter in the column at the far right of the matrix ("Course Total") the number of Sub-competencies reported as receiving major and minor emphasis with reference to each course. Note that these totals reflect the number of 2s and 1s, a frequency count, not the mathematical sum. As you total these counts, include both figures of the "fraction," so that 2/2 adds 4 to the total, whereas 2/0 would add only 2 to the total. Next, total each column vertically and enter that total number in the row marked "Competency Total."

The resulting "Course Total" represents the coverage of all Sub-competencies by course. The highest possible Course Total for each course is 141, which is the total number of entry-level Sub-competencies in the HESPA Model.

The "Competency Total" represents the coverage of each Sub-competency across all courses in the curriculum. This highest possible Competency Total for each Sub-competency is dependent upon the number of courses in the curricula. For example, the four Sub-competencies in Competency 1.1 multiplied by 10 courses in the curricula would generate a possible total of 40 as the Competency Total for that Sub-competency.

Appendix D: Competency Matrices

Analysis Sheet: Areas of Responsibility

Entry-level

Area →	Area I							Area II					Area III				Area IV							Area V							Area VI			Area VII				Course Total^
Competency →	1.1	1.2	1.3	1.4	1.5	1.6	1.7	2.1	2.2	2.3	2.4	2.5	3.1	3.2	3.3	3.4	4.1	4.2	4.3	4.4	4.5	4.6	4.7	5.1	5.2	5.3	5.4	5.5	5.6	6.1	6.2	6.3	7.1	7.2	7.3	7.4	
# Sub-competencies	4	5	5	3	4	5	4	5	5	7	9	2	6	1	6	8	0	0	2	3	0	0	4	0	4	4	4	5	1	5	0	0	6	9	7	8	
Course Title ↓																																					
Community* Health	2/1	0/1	0/3	0/3	4/0	4/1	2/2																														
Biostatistics	0/3	2/2	0/4	2/1	0/2	0/0	0/1																														
Administration of H.E.	0/0	0/3	1/0	0/1	0/0	5/0	4/0																														
School Health	0/4	0/2	0/3	0/1	4/0	2/3	2/2																														
Competency Total^^ →	10	10	11	8	10	15	13																														
Proposed New Courses																																					

*Top number: Number of Sub-competencies given major emphasis (number of "2s" in Area of Responsibility Matrix);
Bottom number: Number of Sub-competencies given minor emphasis (number of "1s" in Area of Responsibility Matrix)
^ Course Total: Sum of top and bottom numbers across all Sub-competencies for the course; Maximum possible course score = 141 (total number of existing Sub-competencies for Entry level)
^^ Competency Total: Sum of top and bottom numbers for all courses for designated Competency; Maximum possible Competency score = # of Sub-competencies x # of courses

Figure D.2 Example Analysis Sheet for Areas of Responsibility

Appendix D: Competency Matrices

Purpose of the Matrices and Analysis Sheets

The matrices and analysis sheets previously described can be used by decision-makers to determine the degree to which each course within a curriculum is addressing the Competencies and Sub-competencies of the Seven Areas of Responsibility. This information can be used to validate curricular strengths and identify potential ways in which the curriculum may be further developed or enhanced so that students are equipped with needed professional Competencies.

A completed analysis sheet (Figure D.2) can provide a summary of the balance of Sub-competency emphases within each Competency of the Seven Areas of Responsibility. The top and bottom numbers in each "cell" of the analysis sheet represent that emphasis balance in each course. For example, the School Health course in Figure D.2 contains an emphasis on all four Sub-competencies in Competency 1.1, but the level of emphasis for all four Sub-competencies is minor, as indicated by the bottom number being a "4" (all scores of 1) and the top number being a "0" (no scores of 2).

The Competency Totals at the bottom of the analysis sheet can be used to identify Sub-competencies that are emphasized the most and least across the curriculum. The Course Totals in the far right column of the sheet can be used to identify the courses in which most Sub-competencies are identified. These two variables are useful in efforts to achieve a balanced approach to Sub-competency emphasis across the curriculum.

The Area of Responsibility matrices (Figure D.1) can provide more details about emphasis levels for each Sub-competency in each course. This information can be useful in determining whether emphasis levels are appropriate in specific courses. If, for example, the community health course was previously designated by decision-makers as the course within the curriculum where at least some emphasis on assessment concepts should be made, a larger number of zeros (0) or ones (1) in the row for that course within the Area I (assessment) matrix could warrant a need for discussion about whether more emphasis for those Sub-competencies in that course is needed. The matrix also can be used to quickly note emphasis levels across courses for a Sub-competency, with the discovery of a large number of zeros or ones in a specific Sub-competency column possibly warrant discussion.

Adapting Existing Curricula

The Curriculum Decision-Making Matrix in Figure D.3 contains a list of questions faculty members may use to summarize findings and determine any necessary actions. It is possible that existing courses in a traditional professional preparation program in health education would not have to be significantly changed to adopt a Competency-based plan. Rather, a need for a new perspective on course goals and objectives and increased use of experiential teaching-learning methods to address the Competency-based Model would be more likely. All of the Competencies for each Area of Responsibility should be included in some instructional activity in a course.

The whole faculty should engage in curriculum design and analysis to enhance consistency in how the Sub-competencies are addressed across the curriculum. Each faculty member responsible for a course should be charged with making any revisions needed to better the fit between course objectives and designated Sub-competencies. All faculty members should participate in planning and designing any new courses deemed necessary to emphasize Sub-competencies currently overlooked. Though knowledge items are not currently used in curriculum analyses, the verified knowledge items in Section VI of this document may be useful in course development.

Appendix D: Competency Matrices

Curriculum Decision-Making Matrix		
Question	Findings	Needed Action
1. How many of the Competencies are currently being addressed by the curriculum?		
2. How many of the Sub-competencies receive major emphasis in the program, as shown by a rating of 2?		
3. How many of the Sub-competencies receive at least minor study, as shown by a rating of 1?		
4. If there are Competencies not now receiving any attention at all, which are they, and in what Area(s) are they found?		
5. In each of the Areas of Responsibility, how many Sub-competencies are not being addressed?		
6. Which courses are providing broadest coverage and which are providing least coverage of the Seven Areas of Responsibility?		
7. Are there any Areas of Responsibility that now receive little if any consideration in the curriculum? If so, which ones?		
8. Are there courses that appear to be irrelevant to the Competencies, as reflected in the number of zeros shown? If so, could this be changed without giving up the course itself?		
9. What implications do you see in these data for course revision, course modification, or the development of new courses?		

Figure D.3 Sample Questions for Curriculum Decision-Making

Appendix D: Competency Matrices

Developing New Curricula

Individuals charged with developing a new curriculum for health education specialists that did not previously exist should begin with the professional preparation curriculum recommended by national health education leaders or by examining curricula of accredited programs. A careful examination of the Sub-competencies across all Seven Areas of Responsibility and discussions with national leaders in program accreditation is recommended prior to curriculum development. The verified knowledge items described in Section VI will be useful in this effort.

In arriving at decisions about where a Competency is to be taught, it is advisable to take an experimental approach. That is, decisions reached at this point need to be regarded as tentative and subject to change through trial and evaluation by students, faculty members, alumni, advisory groups, and employers of program graduates. Several years of evaluation and modification may be necessary before there is assurance that the curriculum is providing opportunities for optimal Competency development. The faculty members also should note that the Competency framework for health education specialists is updated through national studies on a regular basis to ensure that the Competency Model used to frame curricula accurately reflects professional practice.

Selecting Teaching-Learning Strategies

It is not the function of a curriculum framework to specify or describe learning opportunities or lesson plans. But rather, a curriculum framework outlines what should be taught—not how to teach it. It is the responsibility of those who deliver the curriculum to select the strategies to be used. Criteria for the selection of a teaching strategy include the following: (a) it must provide practice in the skill specified in the objective; (b) it must arrange for the discovery or introduction of the content; (c) the activities must be satisfying to the learner; and (d) the activities must be appropriate to the past experiences and present abilities of the learner. If several strategies meet the preceding criteria, the one chosen should be the strategy most likely to produce more than one positive outcome. In general, experiential learning is more effective than passive learning in promoting competency. That is, most people learn better by doing than by watching or listening. The best teaching-learning strategy is the one that provides the learners with a sound understanding of the concept being taught and encourages learners to practice doing what the objective proposes what they need to be competent.

The Competency Framework by Areas of Responsibility

Each of the Seven Areas of Responsibility constituting the Competency-based curriculum framework is introduced by a discussion of each area in Section III. In that section, a general statement is provided that describes each of the Areas of Responsibility in terms of its purpose, meaning, application in health education practice, and relation to the other areas.

The Competency framework for each Area is developed hierarchically as a set of Competency statements, each of which is supported by more specific and narrowly drawn Sub-competencies, upon which measurable general objectives are based and proposed. The sequence in which the Areas of Responsibility is presented is more or less logical, but not absolute. No priorities are intended, nor should any be presumed.

Appendix D: Competency Matrices

Area of Responsibility I Matrix
Area I: Assess Needs, Resources, and Capacity for Health Education/Promotion

Entry-level

Course Title	Comp 1.1 Sub-comp					Comp 1.2 Sub-comp						Comp 1.3 Sub-comp					Comp 1.4 Sub-comp			Comp 1.5 Sub-comp				Comp 1.6 Sub-comp					Comp 1.7 Sub-comp					Total by Course (Max=60)*
	.1	.2	.3	.4	.5	.1	.2	.3	.4	.5	.6	.1	.2	.3	.4	.5	.1	.2	.3	.1	.2	.3	.4	.1	.2	.3	.4	.5	.2	.3	.4	.5	

Total by Area of Responsibility*
Should not exceed maximum (60) x number of courses

Advanced 1-level

Course Title	Comp 1.1 Sub-comp .4	Comp 1.2 Sub-comp .2	Comp 1.7 Sub-comp .1	Total by Course (Max = 6)

Total by Area of Responsibility
Should not exceed maximum (6) x number of courses

Codes: 2=Major Emphasis, 1=Minor Emphasis, 0=No Emphasis
*Max: Maximum number possible per course
^No advanced 2-level Sub-competencies exist for Area of Responsibility I

Figure D.4 Area of Responsibility I Matrix

Appendix D: Competency Matrices

Area of Responsibility II Matrix
Area II: Plan Health Education/Promotion

Entry-level

Course Title	Comp 2.1 Sub-comp					Comp 2.2 Sub-comp					Comp 2.3 Sub-comp									Comp 2.4 Sub-comp										Comp 2.5 Sub-Comp		Total by Course (Max=56)*
	.1	.2	.3	.4	.5	.1	.2	.3	.4	.5	.1	.2	.3	.4	.5	.6	.7	.8	.9	.10	.11	.12	.1	.2	.3	.4	.5	.6	.7	.8	.9	.10	.1	.2	
Total by Area of Responsibility*																																			

Should not exceed maximum (56) x number of courses

Advanced 1-level^

Course Title	Comp 2.3 Sub-comp			Comp 2.4 Sub-comp			Total by Course (Max = 12)
	.1	.2	.3	.8	.9	.10	
Total by Area of Responsibility							

Should not exceed maximum (12) x number of courses

Codes: 2=Major Emphasis, 1=Minor Emphasis, 0=No Emphasis
*Max: Maximum number possible per course
^No advanced 2-level Sub-competencies exist for Area of Responsibility II

Figure D.5 Area of Responsibility II Matrix

Appendix D: Competency Matrices

Area of Responsibility III Matrix
Area III: Implement Health Education/Promotion

Entry-level

Course Title	Comp 3.1 Sub-comp						Comp 3.2 Sub-comp		Comp 3.3 Sub-comp								Comp 3.4 Sub-comp								Total by Course (Max=42)
	.1	.2	.3	.4	.5	.6	.1	.2	.1	.2	.3	.4	.5	.6	.7	.8	.1	.2	.3	.4	.5	.6	.7	.8	

Total by Area of Responsibility

Should not exceed maximum (42) × number of courses

Advanced 1-level^

Course Title	Comp 3.2 Sub-comp								Comp 3.3 Sub-comp		Total by Course (Max = 16)
	.1	.2	.3	.4	.5	.6	.7	.8	.1	.2	

Total by Area of Responsibility

Should not exceed maximum (16) × number of courses

Codes: 2=Major Emphasis, 1=Minor Emphasis, 0=No Emphasis
*Max: Maximum number possible per course
^No advanced 2-level Sub-competencies exist for Area of Responsibility III

Figure D.6 Area of Responsibility III Matrix

Appendix D: Competency Matrices

Area of Responsibility IV Matrix

Area IV: Conduct Evaluation and Research Related to Health Education/Promotion

Entry-level

Course Title	Comp 4.3 Sub-comp					Comp 4.4 Sub-comp					Comp 4.7 Sub-comp				Total by Course (Max=18)
	.1	.2	.3	.4	.5	.3	.4	.5			.1	.2	.3	.4	

Total by Area of Responsibility
Should not exceed maximum (18) x number of courses

Area IV: Advanced 1-level

Course Title	Comp 4.1 Sub-comp										Comp 4.5 Sub-comp		Total by Course (Max=20)*
	.1	.2	.3	.4	.5	.6	.7	.8	.9	.10	.1	.2	

Total by Area of Responsibility
Should not exceed maximum (20) x number of courses

Codes: 2=Major Emphasis, 1=Minor Emphasis, 0=No Emphasis
*Max: Maximum number possible per course

Figure D.7 Area of Responsibility IV Matrix

Appendix D: Competency Matrices

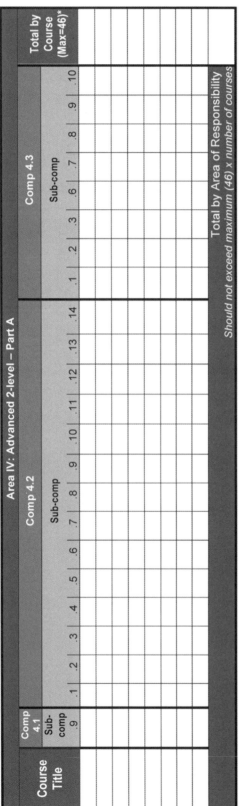

Figure D.7.A Area IV: Advanced 2-level—Part A Matrix

Figure D.7.B Area IV: Advanced 2-level—Part B Matrix

Codes: 2=Major Emphasis, 1=Minor Emphasis, 0=No Emphasis
*Max: Maximum number possible per course

Appendix D: Competency Matrices

Area of Responsibility V Matrix
Area V: Administer and Manage Health Education/Promotion

Entry-level

Course Title	Comp 5.2 Sub-comp						Comp 5.3 Sub-comp					Comp 5.4 Sub-comp				Comp 5.5 Sub-comp				Comp 5.6 Sub-comp	Total by Course (Max = 36)*
	.1	.2	.3	.4	.5	.6	.1	.3	.4	.5	.6	.1	.2	.3	.4	.2	.3	.8	.9	.10	.5

Total by Area of Responsibility (36) x number of courses
Should not exceed maximum

Advanced 1-level^

Course Title	Comp 5.1 Sub-comp														Comp 5.3 Sub-comp	Comp 5.5 Sub-comp				Comp 5.6 Sub-comp						Total by Course (Max = 66)*
	.1	.2	.3	.4	.5	.6	.7	.8	.9	.10	.11	.12	.13	.2	.5	.1	.4	.5	.6	.7	.1	.2	.3	.4	.6	.7	.8	.9	.10	.11	.12	.13	.14

Total by Area of Responsibility (66) x number of courses
Should not exceed maximum

Codes: 2=Major Emphasis, 1=Minor Emphasis, 0=No Emphasis
*Max: Maximum number possible per course
^No advanced 2-level Sub-competencies exist for Area of Responsibility V

Figure D.8 Area of Responsibility V Matrix

Appendix D: Competency Matrices

Area of Responsibility VI Matrix
Area VI: Serve as a Health Education/Promotion Resource Person

Course Title	Comp 6.1 Sub-comp					Total by Course (Max=10)*
	.1	.2	.3	.4	.5	
Total by Area of Responsibility						

Should not exceed maximum (10) x number of courses

Advanced 1-level^

Course Title	Comp 6.2 Sub-comp						Comp 6.3 Sub-comp					Total by Course (Max=22)
	.1	.2	.3	.4	.5	.6	.1	.2	.3	.4	.5	
Total by Area of Responsibility												

Should not exceed maximum (22) x number of courses

Codes: 2=Major Emphasis, 1=Minor Emphasis, 0=No Emphasis
*Max: Maximum number possible per course
^No advanced 2-level Sub-competencies exist for Area of Responsibility VI

Figure D.9 Area of Responsibility VI Matrix

Appendix D: Competency Matrices

Area of Responsibility VII Matrix
Area VII: Communicate, Promote, and Advocate for Health, Health Education/Promotion, and the Profession

Entry-level

Course Title	Comp 7.1 Sub-comp								Comp 7.2 Sub-comp								Comp 7.3 Sub-comp										Comp 7.4 Sub-comp								Total by Course (Max=60)*
	.1	.2	.3	.4	.5	.6	.7	.8	.1	.2	.3	.4	.5	.6	.7	.8	.1	.2	.3	.4	.5	.6	.7	.8	.9	.10	.1	.2	.3	.4	.5	.6	.7	.8	

Should not exceed maximum (60) × number of courses — Total by Area of Responsibility

Advanced 1-level | Advanced 2-level

Course Title	Comp 7.1 Sub-comp		Comp 7.3 Sub-comp			Comp 7.4 Sub-comp			Total by Course (Max=16)*
	.4	.5	.6	.7	.8	.9	.10	.11	

Should not exceed maximum (16) × number of courses — Total by Area of Responsibility

Codes: 2=Major Emphasis, 1=Minor Emphasis, 0=No Emphasis
*Max: Maximum number possible per course

Figure D.10 Area of Responsibility VII Matrix

Appendix D: Competency Matrices

Analysis Sheet: Areas of Responsibility

Entry Level

Area →	Area I								Area II						Area III					Area IV								Area V							Area VI				Area VII				Course Total^
Competency →	1.1	1.2	1.3	1.4	1.5	1.6	1.7		2.1	2.2	2.3	2.4	2.5		3.1	3.2	3.3	3.4		4.1	4.2	4.3	4.4	4.5	4.6	4.7		5.1	5.2	5.3	5.4	5.5	5.6		6.1	6.2	6.3		7.1	7.2	7.3	7.4	
# Sub-competencies →	4	5	5	3	4	5	4		5	5	7	9	2		6	1	6	8		0	0	2	3	0	0	4		0	4	4	4	5	1		5	0	0		6	9	7	8	
Course Title ↓																																											

| Competency Total^^ → | | | | | | | | | | | | | | | | | | | | | | | | | | | | | | | | | | | | | | | | | | | |
| Proposed New Courses | | | | | | | | | | | | | | | | | | | | | | | | | | | | | | | | | | | | | | | | | | | |

*Top number: Number of Sub-competencies given <u>major</u> emphasis *(number of "2s" in Area of Responsibility Matrix)*;
 Bottom number: Number of Sub-competencies given minor emphasis *(number of "1s" in Area of Responsibility Matrix)*
^ Course Total: Sum of top and bottom numbers across all Sub-competencies for the course; *Maximum possible course score* = 141 (total number of existing Sub-competencies for Entry level)
^^ Competency Total: Sum of top and bottom numbers for all courses for designated Competency; *Maximum possible Competency score* = # of Sub-competencies x # of courses

Figure D.11 Analysis Sheet: **Areas of Responsibility, Entry Level**

Appendix D: Competency Matrices

Analysis Sheet: Areas of Responsibility

Advanced 1-level

Area→	Area I								Area II						Area III					Area IV								Area V							Area VI				Area VII				
Competency→	1.1	1.2	1.3	1.4	1.5	1.6	1.7		2.1	2.2	2.3	2.4	2.5		3.1	3.2	3.3	3.4		4.1	4.2	4.3	4.4	4.5	4.6	4.7		5.1	5.2	5.3	5.4	5.5	5.6		6.1	6.2	6.3		7.1	7.2	7.3	7.4	Course Total^
# Sub-competencies→	1	1	0	0	0	0	1		0	0	5	1	0		0	7	1	0		9	0	0	0	1	0	0		13	0	2	0	5	13		0	6	5		2	0	3	0	
Course Title→																																											
Competency Total^^→																																											
Proposed New Courses																																											

*Top number: Number of Sub-competencies given major emphasis *(number of "2s" in Area of Responsibility Matrix)*;
Bottom number: Number of Sub-competencies given minor emphasis *(number of "1s" in Area of Responsibility Matrix)*
^ Course Total: Sum of top and bottom numbers across all Sub-competencies for the course; *Maximum possible course score* = 76 (total number of existing Sub-competencies for Advanced 1-level)
^^ Competency Total: Sum of top and bottom numbers for all courses for designated Competency: *Maximum possible Competency score* = # of Sub-competencies x # of courses

Figure D.12 Analysis Sheet; Areas of Responsibility, Advanced 1-level

Appendix D: Competency Matrices

Analysis Sheet: Areas of Responsibility
Advanced 2-level

Area →	Area IV						Area VII	Course Total^
Competency →	4.1	4.2	4.3	4.4	4.5	4.6	4.7	7.4	
# Sub-competencies →	1	14	8	2	4	8	1	3	
Course Title ↓									

Competency Total^^ →									
Proposed New Courses									

*Areas of Responsibility I, II, III, V, and VI do not contain Advanced 2-level Sub-competencies **Top number: Number of Sub-competencies given major emphasis (*number of "2s" in Area of Responsibility Matrix*) ^ **Course Total:** Sum of top and bottom numbers across all Sub-competencies for Advanced 2-level)
Bottom number: Number of Sub-competencies given minor emphasis (*number of "1s" in Area of Responsibility Matrix*)
Maximum possible course score = 41 (total number of existing Sub-competencies for Advanced 2-level)
^^ **Competency Total:** Sum of top and bottom numbers for all courses for designated Competency; *Maximum possible Competency score* = # of Sub-competencies x # of courses

***Figure D.13** Analysis Sheet: Areas of Responsibility, Advanced 2-level*